D Giblin

AN ABC OF ENDOCRINOLOGY

K. J. CATT

M.D., Ph.D., F.R.A.C.P.

Visiting Scientist, Reproduction Research Branch,
National Institute for Child Health and Human Development,
National Institutes of Health, Bethesda, Maryland,
and Associate Clinical Professor of Medicine,
Georgetown University, Georgetown, Washington, D.C.

LITTLE, BROWN AND COMPANY
BOSTON

LIBRARY OF CONGRESS CATALOG CARD NO. 70–160740

FIRST EDITION

Second Printing

ISBN 0–316–13190

MOST OF THIS MONOGRAPH FIRST APPEARED AS A SERIES OF ARTICLES IN THE LANCET. PUBLICATION IN BOOK FORM INCORPORATES ADDITIONAL MATERIAL AND ILLUSTRATIONS.

Published in Great Britain
by The Lancet Ltd., London

PRINTED IN THE UNITED STATES OF AMERICA

Contents

CHAPTER ONE
Hormones in General   1

CHAPTER TWO
Pituitary Function   9

CHAPTER THREE
Growth Hormone   21

CHAPTER FOUR
Reproductive Endocrinology   40

CHAPTER FIVE
Adrenal Cortex   60

CHAPTER SIX
The Thyroid Gland   82

CHAPTER SEVEN
Hormonal Control of Calcium Homœostasis   98

CHAPTER EIGHT
Insulin and Glucose Homœostasis   106

CHAPTER NINE
Endocrine Changes During Pregnancy   122

CHAPTER TEN
Endocrine-Function Tests   137

Glossary   148

Index   149

Introduction

DURING the past few years, fresh insights into the synthesis, secretion, metabolism, and action of hormones have resulted from the applications of new techniques for the investigation of basic and clinical endocrine problems. Improved methods for purification and radio-labelling of peptide and protein hormones have enabled measurement of these molecules in plasma to be performed down to the nanogramme and picogramme range. The mode of action of hormones at the cell level has been widely explored through studies on the localisation and intracellular actions of steroid hormones and by extensive studies on the role of cyclic nucleotides as intracellular mediators of peptide-hormone action. Progress has been rapid in many other areas of endocrine research—notably in the structural analysis and synthesis of peptide hormones—and clinical applications have been close behind.

In the following chapters, reprinted from a successful series in *The Lancet*, Dr. Catt surveys current knowledge of hormone secretion and actions, with particular attention to information gained from recent research. Two chapters have been added—one an account of endocrine changes in pregnancy, the other a brief description of the tests used to assess endocrine function.

The following figures are reproduced by permission of the authors and publishers: fig. 6 (Dr. S. Glick and Excerpta Medica), fig. 11 (Dr. V. Stevens and Lippincott), fig. 12 (Dr. R. Midgley and Lippincott), fig. 14 (Dr. G. Ross and Lippincott), fig. 18 (Dr. R. Peterson and Macmillan), and fig. 25 (Dr. D. Fawcett and Academic Press). The following figures have been modified, with permission, from published material: fig. 1 (Dr. B. O'Malley and Academic Press), fig. 2 (Dr. C. Sawin and Little, Brown), fig. 4 (Dr. D. Fawcett and Academic Press), fig. 27 (Dr. J. Potts and Saunders), fig. 28 (Dr. D. H. Copp and Excerpta Medica), and fig. 29 (Dr. H. DeLuca and Excerpta Medica).

Editor of *The Lancet.*

CHAPTER ONE

Hormones in General

THE endocrine system consists of a diverse group of tissues with the common property of producing chemical stimuli to other tissues, and secreting these into the circulation. Starling's original use of the term "hormone" to describe secretin and gastrin was followed by its application to the secretions of the pituitary and its end-organs, and of the parathyroids, pancreatic islet-cells, and placenta. This classical group of hormones has now been supplemented by the components of the renin-angiotensin system and by several new peptide hormones such as calcitonin and placental lactogen. Finally, the gut hormones have been further confirmed as such by the recognition of their role in insulin secretion.

Hormones are usually secreted into the circulation in extremely low concentration, and mostly are recognised only by specific tissues which respond in characteristic fashion. The plasma concentration of steroid and thyroid hormones ranges between 10^{-6} and $10^{-9}M$ and peptide hormones between 10^{-10} and $10^{-12}M$ (compared with about $10^{-1}M$ for sodium, $10^{-2}M$ for glucose, and $10^{-3}M$ for albumin). Moreover, in the end-organs the cellular response to hormone stimulation is usually restricted: the trophic hormones cause the production of secondary hormones such as thyroxine or cortisol, with more diverse effects on cellular metabolism in other tissues. By contrast, the gonadal steroids exert their effects on several responsive tissues.

The definition of a hormone should not be confined to substances secreted by a recognisable endocrine organ. Some hormones, such as angiotensin II, are formed from precursors in the circulation; others are formed by conversion from precursors in tissues, such as testosterone in the female and dihydrotestosterone in many androgen-responsive cells. Therefore the actions, as well as the origins, of blood-borne stimuli should be considered when deciding whether or not such stimuli should be classed as hormones. Whatever their origin, hormones do not themselves take part in energy-producing processes, but exert profound regulatory effects upon the growth, differentiation, and metabolic activity of many tissues.

Hormone Action

The primary event of hormone action is the specific interaction between hormone and responsive cell. Many cells do not recognise certain hormones; hence the receptor sites of the cell membrane must be highly specific. Few hormones exert any detectable effect when added directly to cell-free systems, and it seems certain that hormone action usually begins at the cell membrane. Earlier theories on hormone action included the regulation of enzyme activity, and the transport mechanisms for small molecules in membranes. Since 1964 most of the known hormones have been found to regulate the synthesis of protein and R.N.A. This has led to the suggestion that hormones may activate genes and cause transcription of new species of messenger R.N.A., which then code for the synthesis of specific proteins. Important evidence for this hypothesis has been provided by study of the actions of œstradiol on the rat uterus[1] and of progesterone and œstradiol on the chick oviduct.[2] Many of the data have been derived from experiments in which the actions of antimetabolites such as actinomycin D (which blocks synthesis of messenger and ribosomal R.N.A.) and puromycin or cycloheximide (which block protein synthesis) have been utilised to determine the step at which the hormone acts (fig. 1); but these toxic inhibitors are not completely specific in their actions, and their effects must be carefully interpreted.

The use of tritium-labelled steroid hormones has revealed specific binding receptors for œstradiol, progesterone, and aldosterone in responsive tissues—uterus, oviduct, and kidney respectively—and autoradiography shows nuclear localisation of labelled steroid in these tissues. The specific association of the steroid hormone with a macromolecular binding protein is a necessary preliminary to its action at a nuclear effector site on the genome, leading to stimulation of R.N.A. transcription.

The role of the cell membrane in hormone action has been further elucidated by the demonstration that 3′5′ cyclic adenosine monophosphate (A.M.P.) apparently mediates the action of many peptide and protein hormones.[3] The adenyl-cyclase system, which is located on the inner surface of cell membranes, catalyses the conversion of adenosine triphosphate (A.T.P.) to cyclic A.M.P. Cyclic A.M.P. has now been shown to be directly involved in the actions of adrenocorticotrophic hormone (A.C.T.H., corticotrophin), luteinising hormone (L.H.), thyroid-stimulating hormone (T.S.H.), melanocyte-stimulating hormone (M.S.H.), antidiuretic hormone (A.D.H.), glucagon, parathyroid hormone, insulin, thyroxine, adrenaline, serotonin, and histamine. Most of these hormones seem to function by stimulating the

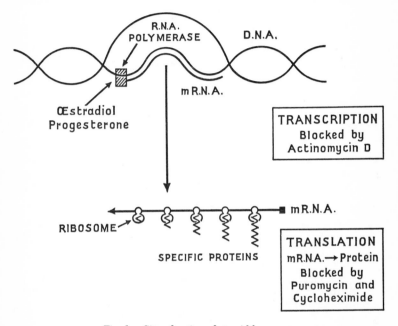

Fig. 1.—*Site of action of steroid hormones.*
Œstradiol and progesterone have been shown to act by modifying nuclear gene expression (transcription). (Modified from O'Malley et al.[2] Copyright Academic Press.)

action of adenyl cyclase, but some may function by inhibiting the phosphodiesterase which degrades cyclic A.M.P. to 5′ A.M.P. (fig. 2).

Sutherland et al.[3] have suggested that cyclic A.M.P. is a "second messenger" propagating through the cell the message brought by the "first messenger", which is the hormone itself. Steroid hormones may be regarded as "third messengers", since their synthesis and secretion are stimulated in several tissues by cyclic A.M.P. Further, second messengers besides cyclic A.M.P. have been supposed to exist: possibly prostaglandins have this function, mediating hormonal inhibition either directly or by blocking formation of cyclic A.M.P.

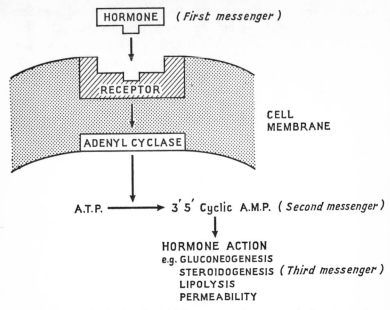

Fig. 2—Proposed role of cyclic A.M.P. as a second messenger for hormone action. The specificity of the hormonal response depends on the existence of unique receptors in the cell membrane. (Modified from Sawin.[4])

In summary, there is now good evidence that steroid hormones act by combining with specific nuclear receptors and modifying the process of gene transcription which leads to R.N.A. formation and protein synthesis. For peptide hormones, the ubiquitous cyclic A.M.P. seems to be an intracellular messenger, transmitting the specific message which has been received and decoded by the interaction of the hormone with the cell membrane. A link between these two systems has been established by the observation that progesterone increases cyclic-A.M.P. formation, and that cyclic A.M.P. itself can affect gene transcription and translation.[2] The nature of the regulatory interactions between hormones and cell components and the mechanisms of hormone action are just beginning to be defined.

Physiological Regulation of Hormonal Activity

All endocrine secretions appear to play a large part in regulating cellular metabolism and functions, and in controlling the physiological responses of the organism. To the biologist hormones are central factors in metabolic, growth, and reproductive processes. To the clinician they are the basis of discrete syndromes of hormonal over-secretion or undersecretion, which usually require endocrine-gland ablation or hormonal replacement therapy. The restoration of normal metabolic function by simple replacement therapy with certain hormones suggests that the presence of hormone concentration above a certain level is more important than the exact circulating concentration. Thus, replacement therapy with thyroxine, cortisol, and growth hormone achieves satisfactory results when a certain minimum level is maintained in body-fluids. Though severe stresses often require concomitant increase in hormone secretion or administration, there is no recognised requirement to mimic the minute-to-minute pattern of endogenous hormone secretion. On the other hand, the control of cyclic functions—for example, the menstrual cycle—calls more clearly for critical hormone levels at critical times; and similar fluctuations are observed in the levels of other hormones concerned with homœostatic adjustment, such as insulin, the gut hormones, and aldosterone.

Hormone secretion must be subject to control mechanisms; in many cases a fairly constant blood-level is required, and some form of sensing device must exist to monitor either the hormone level itself or some related function such as plasma osmolality, blood-glucose, or body-sodium content. Negative feedback is a common control mechanism for hormone secretion, particularly in the secretion of pituitary trophic hormones in response to peripheral hormone levels. In this form of control, the effects of a hormone reduce further secretion of the hormone. The products of pituitary trophic hormones (cortisol, thyroxine, gonadal steroids) feed back on the hypothalamus and pituitary, depressing the secretion of further trophic hormone. Similarly, parathyroid hormone and insulin are secreted in accordance with negative feedback from serum-calcium and blood-glucose levels. Negative-feedback systems are generally more complex than this description indicates, sometimes operating indirectly via several steps, sometimes involving more than one action of the feedback hormone—e.g., œstradiol inhibits secretion of follicle-stimulating hormone (F.S.H.) and stimulates release of L.H. In addition, non-hormonal and environmental factors may alter the feed-back control system or its response. Nevertheless, negative-feedback control remains central to notions about hormone secretion and provides a rational basis for interpreting and managing clinical syndromes. Positive feedback, wherein the hormone further stimulates the events leading to its own secretion, is much less common and may be exemplified by the relation between œstradiol and luteinising-hormone release before ovulation.

Endocrine Investigation

Being potent and transient messengers, hormones are usually secreted rapidly in response to a stimulus, circulate in extremely low concentration, and are metabolised at rates roughly related to the speed of their regulated function—e.g., corticosteroids in hours, angiotensin II, A.C.T.H., and insulin in minutes. Because the levels of hormone and hormonal metabolites in body fluids are so low, laboratory methodology has always figured prominently in endocrine investigations and research. In addition many of the important stimuli to basic endocrine research have come from clinical observations on hormonal experiments of Nature. Formerly, disordered physiology was the major preoccupation of the endocrinologist; but latterly he has been more concerned with the biochemical lesion underlying the disturbance of function.

Measurement of hormones in blood is usually preferable to measurement in urine. Estimates of urinary hormone excretion may usefully reflect total hormone secretion, but the development of specific methods to measure the production-rates of hormones has given much more precise estimates. Single measurements of urine or blood levels of a hormone, or even of secretion-rates, do not always suffice to exclude malfunction of the gland concerned; in addition, measurement of levels or secretion-rates before and during steps to stimulate or suppress the gland may be necessary. Thus, in the assessment of suspected pituitary, adrenal, thyroid, and gonadal hypofunction, stimulation tests by induced metabolic disturbances or administration of trophic hormones may be necessary to evaluate the extent of the disorder. Conversely, suppression tests may be necessary to confirm the autonomous hypersecretion of hormones that occurs in acromegaly, thyrotoxicosis, Conn's syndrome, and sometimes in Cushing's syndrome.

Subtle disorders of steroid hormone secretion are not now believed to be common causes of potentially related disorders such as diabetes mellitus and hypertension. Conversely, the physical changes which do result from long-standing hormone excess, such as the hypertension of Conn's syndrome, the hirsutism of androgen excess, and the functional hypothalamic lesion of glucocorticoid excess, are known sometimes to persist long after the hypersecretion has been corrected.

New Hormones

Since 1960 several new hormones, mainly of peptide or protein nature, have been described. These include two placental hormones with certain similarities to pituitary hormones—human placental lactogen (H.P.L.) with immunological and structural features in common with human growth hormone (H.G.H.), and a placental thyrotrophic protein. From the sheep pituitary a lipotrophic peptide has been identified and characterised, and a comparable lipotrophic peptide has been described in association with H.G.H. in man. The structural analysis and synthesis of several gut hormones such as gastrin, secretin, glucagon, and cholecystokinin have been achieved; and the discovery, isolation, sequence determination, and synthesis of calcitonin have been performed during the relatively short period of seven years. The hypothalamic hormones controlling pituitary function have also been characterised, and a thyrotrophin-releasing tripeptide has been synthesised. By contrast, it is now recognised that in thyrotoxicosis thyroid function is stimulated, not by thyrotrophin as under normal circumstances, but apparently by an abnormal stimulator with the characteristics of γ-globulin.

In addition to these newly described protein hormones, secretion of hormonal peptides from ectopic sites has been recognised to occur in certain tumours, mainly those arising in tissues of foregut origin.[6] The ectopic hormone syndromes have been most commonly observed in lung tumours and have included the secretion of A.C.T.H., antidiuretic hormone, growth hormone, H.P.L., gonadotrophins, and parathyroid hormone. Most of the peptide hormones are normally secreted from tissues which originate from the alimentary tract during embryonic development—i.e., pituitary, thyroid-parathyroid, and islet-cells.

Among the steroid hormones, the major newcomer has been dihydrotestosterone, a reduced form of testosterone which seems likely to be the active androgenic hormone at the tissue level. Also, the secretion of conjugated steroids, such as dehydroepiandrosterone sulphate from the adrenal, has been recognised to occur. These and other steroids may function as prehormones, leading to the production of active hormones in blood or tissue by metabolism or interconversion from a relatively less active precursor molecule.

Measurement of Hormones

The methods used in endocrine research and diagnosis have been considerably expanded by the application of techniques from cytogenetics, immunology, protein chemistry, and electron microscopy. Chemical assay has almost completely replaced bioassay in most areas of endocrine research, though in gonadotrophin estimations new techniques such as radioimmunoassay have been used to complement bioassay, rather than to supersede the older procedures. There remains a great need for ultrasensitive bioassay procedures, based on such indicators as radioactive substrates or induced enzyme changes, to allow further investigation of protein-hormone effects in vivo, and eventually to be superseded by even more subtle and sensitive chemical assays. Considerable activity in endocrine research is now being directed towards the chemical, physical, and immunological estimation of hormones and their metabolites and the eiucidation of the structure, metabolism, and actions of peptide and protein hormones. Much is known about the structure and metabolism of steroid hormones, and current investigation is concerned with their biosynthesis, control of secretion, and mechanism of action.

1. Gorski, J., Noteboom, W. D., Nicolette, J. A. *J. cell. comp. Physiol.* 1965, **66**, suppl. 1, 91.
2. O'Malley, B. W., McGuire, W. L., Kohler, P. O., Korenman, S. G. *Rec. Prog. Horm. Res.* 1969, **25**, 105.
3. Sutherland, E. W., Øye, I., Butcher, R. W. *ibid.* 1965, **21**, 623.
4. Sawin, C. T. The Hormones. Boston, 1969.
5. Munck, A. *in* Recent Advances in Endocrinology (edited by V. H. T. James); p. 139. Boston, 1968.
6. Liddle, G. W., Nicholson, W. F., Island, D. P., Orth, D. O., Abe, K., Lowder, S. C. *Rec. Prog. Horm. Res.* 1969, **25**, 283.

CHAPTER TWO

Pituitary Function

MOST of the peptide and glycoprotein hormones secreted by the anterior pituitary gland are trophic hormones—A.C.T.H., T.S.H., F.S.H., L.H.—which stimulate the secretory activity of peripheral endocrine tissues such as adrenals, thyroid, and gonads. The pituitary also secretes growth hormone (G.H.) and lipotrophic hormone, which exert direct metabolic effects upon tissues, and M.S.H., which does not have a clearcut function in man. The end-results of pituitary hormone secretion are concerned either with metabolic regulation (G.H., A.C.T.H., T.S.H.) or with reproduction (L.H., F.S.H., prolactin).

Regulation of Anterior-pituitary Function

Three mechanisms are involved in the control of anterior-pituitary hormone secretion: (i) information transfer from the hypothalamus by local hormones with specific effects upon pituitary hormone release, (ii) feedback by the products of the endocrine target organ, and (iii) feedback by the pituitary hormones themselves. The hypothalamic mechanism stimulates all pituitary hormones except prolactin and M.S.H., which it inhibits. Feedback by adrenal steroids, sex steroids, and thyroid hormones inhibits the release of the respective trophic hormones, with the exception of œstrogen, which can stimulate L.H. release by positive feedback. The feedback by pituitary hormones themselves is not yet fully understood.

Hypothalamic Control[1-4]

The blood-supply to the anterior pituitary gland is almost completely derived from the portal system which arises in the primary capillary plexus of the median eminence and neural stalk. Within the pituitary, the portal system divides into sinusoids, the cells of the gland being separated from the blood only by endothelium and a perisinusoidal space. This arrangement provides a pathway for the control of pituitary secretion by transmitters released from terminals adjacent to the capillary loops in the median eminence. These transmitter molecules have been termed "releasing factors", but "hypo-thalamic neurohormones" is a more general description, indicating both the origin and the hormonal nature of the transmitter molecules, and including both releasing factors (R.F.) and inhibiting factors (I.F.). Most of the hypothalamic neurohormones are stimulatory in action, including growth-hormone-releasing factor (G.H.R.F.), luteinising-hormone-releasing factor (L.H.R.F.), follicle-stimulating-hormone-releasing factor (F.S.H.R.F.) thyroid-stimulating-hormone-releasing factor (T.S.H.R.F., T.R.F.), and corticotrophin-releasing factor (C.R.F.). In two cases, prolactin and M.S.H., the neurohormones have an inhibitory effect and are termed prolactin-inhibiting factor (P.I.F.) and melanocyte-inhibiting factor (M.I.F.). The immediate control of the secretory activity of anterior pituitary cells is by stimulation or inhibition of hormone synthesis and release by these local hormones arising in the adjacent hypothalamus. The hypothalamic hormones are themselves formed at the terminals of axons originating in areas of the hypothalamus concerned with integration of feedback by peripheral hormones, metabolic stimuli, and neural influences.

The existence of hypophysiotrophic areas in the hypothalamus has been established by study of the effects of localised stimulation, localised lesions, and hormone implantation, but the functions of these areas do not correspond precisely with the anatomical nuclei of the hypothalamus. Control of A.C.T.H. secretion appears to be localised in the posterior hypothalamus, control of T.S.H. in the anterior part, gonadotrophin control in the anterior and middle regions, and H.G.H. control in a large area of the ventral hypothalamus.

The long portal vessels which originate in the median eminence supply the lateral and inferior aspects of the pituitary and carry the major part of the gland's blood-supply. There is also a group of short portal vessels which run between the lower part of the pituitary stalk and the upper part of the gland, supplying about 10% of the pituitary and possibly maintaining the viability of part of the gland following stalk section. Individual portal vessels probably supply fairly discrete segments of pituitary tissue.

Hormones of the Hypothalamus

The hypothalamic regulator hormones, which specifically stimulate the release of A.C.T.H., T.S.H., G.H., L.H., and F.S.H. from the pituitary and inhibit the release of prolactin and M.S.H., are all of low molecular weight (from a few hundred to 2000) and are active in minute concentrations (a few nanogrammes will produce an effect on in-vitro assay systems employing pituitary tissue). The chemical nature of these hormones has been difficult to determine, since the yields from hypothalamic tissue are extremely small. T.S.H.R.F. (or T.R.F.) is a tripeptide ([pyr]-glu-his-pro[NH2$_2$]) which has been synthesised and shown to cause T.S.H. release in animals and man; G.H.R.F. and L.H.R.F. are also known to be small peptides, containing about 10 aminoacid residues. These have also been shown to cause release of their respective trophic hormones in vitro and in vivo, while porcine L.H.R.F. has been shown to stimulate gonadotrophin release in man as well as in other species including rabbit, rat, monkey, and sheep. Purified and synthetic L.H.R.F. preparations cause release of both L.H. and F.S.H. from the pituitary, so a degree of F.S.H.-releasing activity is intrinsic to the L.H.R.F. molecule. The chemical natures of P.I.F. and M.I.F. are unknown.

The hypothalamic hormones are primarily concerned with regulation of hormone secretion by stimulation or inhibition of release. Effects upon synthesis of hormones have not yet been fully explored, though it is likely that G.H.R.F. stimulates synthesis as well as release of G.H.

Negative-feedback Control of Pituitary Function (fig. 3)

The hormones produced by the adrenals, gonads, and thyroid in response to pituitary trophic hormones feed back to the hypothalamus and pituitary and reduce the secretion of trophic hormones. Changes in blood-levels of adrenal and gonadal hormones are monitored by hypothalamic receptors, modifying the synthesis of releasing hormones and thereby causing appropriate changes in trophic-hormone secretion. In this way, the peripheral levels of the steroid hormones are kept constant, or within the set limits of cyclical variations. In T.S.H. secretion, feedback by thyroid hormones occurs mainly at the pituitary level. There is no clearcut feedback control system for G.H. apart from the inhibiting effect of glucose on G.H. release via the hypothalamus.

As well as these long feedback loops involving peripheral hormones or metabolic factors there are also short feedback loops by which pituitary hormones can reflexly modify their own rate of secretion by acting back directly upon the hypothalamus. There is evidence for autoregulation of A.C.T.H., L.H., and F.S.H., and probably also for

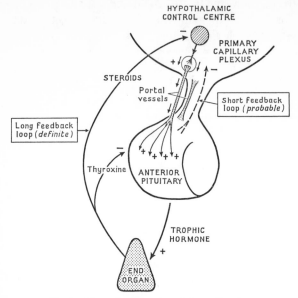

Fig. 3—Control of anterior pituitary function.

Releasing hormones are secreted into the primary capillary plexus of the portal vessels and pass along them to stimulate trophic-hormone release by the cells of the anterior pituitary. Negative feedback occurs from peripheral hormones (long loop) and trophic hormones (short loop) to the hypothalamus.

G.H. and M.S.H. A short-loop control system could prevent wide variations in trophic-hormone secretion, whereas the long-loop feedback by peripheral hormones would adjust the overall secretion-rates according to metabolic demands and reproductive rhythms. A possible avenue for the short feedback is provided by the short portal vessels, which might carry a sample of the pituitary blood back to the pituitary stalk and adjacent hypothalamus. Small quantities of A.C.T.H., L.H., and F.S.H. have been detected in hypothalamic extracts.

Central-nervous-system Control of Pituitary Activity

The hypothalamic neurohormones allow anterior-pituitary function to be substantially influenced by other areas of the central nervous system. The widespread neural connections of the hypothalamus with the limbic system, globus pallidus, and forebrain are involved in the neuroendocrine responses to homœostatic and reproductive demands. Lesions or stimuli in these regions can modify pituitary hormone secretion, in particular by interfering with the intrinsic cycles responsible for diurnal variations in pituitary secretion. The electrical activity of the limbic and hypothalamic areas can be modified by gonadal steroids and antifertility agents, and also by glucocorticoids and stress. These interrelations between the endocrine system and the central nervous system, obviously important for the integrated regulation of hormonal secretion in meeting internal requirements, are equally important in controlling the response to environmental and emotional stimuli. Such responses are most clearly important in two sometimes related areas of activity—stress and reproduction. The integrated neuroendocrine response to stress, with associated secretion of catecholamines and A.C.T.H., is well known, and environmental stimuli—light, sound, and smell—have been shown to influence reproductive behaviour and function in mammals.[5]

Responses to environmental stimuli are of three types:

(i) A rapid response mediated directly through the central nervous system (e.g., visual or olfactory cues in sexual behaviour) or through neurohumoral channels involving the posterior pituitary (e.g., the milk-ejection-reflex response to suckling).

(ii) A delayed response, dependent upon the anterior pituitary and characteristic of the exteroceptive stimulation (e.g., effects of odour on œstrus and pregnancy; effects of seasonal light variations on reproductive function).

(iii) Imprinting, the permanent modification of behaviour resulting from stimulation at a critical period of development.

The effects of light have been attributed to the synthesis of melatonin by the pineal gland. Stimuli from the retina pass via the cervical sympathetic system to the pineal and influence the activity of a rate-limiting enzyme concerned with melatonin synthesis. In some species melatonin inhibits ovarian function and development.[6] These effects of light are important mainly for seasonal variation in reproductive function.

Odours greatly influence reproductive function in many mammals.[5] In female mice the odour of a male will stimulate gonadotrophin release, œstrus, and ovulation, whereas the presence of other females suppresses œstrus. If a mated female mouse is exposed to other males before implantation has occurred the pregnancy is blocked by inhibition of prolactin secretion, which is again due to the odour of the male. Sexual preferences in female mice seem to originate in imprinting by early olfactory experiences such as exposure to male odour during rearing.

Sexual Differentiation of the Hypothalamus[7]

The rhythmic release of gonadotrophin from the pituitary during œstrus and the menstrual cycle is controlled by an interplay between the hypothalamus, pituitary, and gonad. The hypothalamus appears to have an endogenous rhythm of hormone release which plays a major part in controlling the reproductive cycle. This programmed activity is characteristic of the female hypothalamus, and is absent in the male. The intrinsic rhythmicity of the hypothalamus for gonadotrophin release is suppressed in male rats by the presence of the testis, and castration of newborn males results in rhythmic gonadotrophin release and the development of growth and behaviour patterns more characteristic of the female. Conversely, testis transplants and androgen treatment in newborn female rats abolish the rhythm and lead to tonic rather than cyclic release of gonadotropins, causing infertility and polycystic ovaries analogous to the Stein-Leventhal syndrome in human beings. Permanent changes in hypothalamic function have also been observed after thyroxine and steroid administration in infant rats.

The critical period for androgen differentiation of the hypothalamus appears to be much earlier in man and most other species than in the rat.

Pituitary Cells and Hormones

Cell Types

The various secretory cells of the pituitary have been identified by staining, immunofluorescence, and electron microscopy.[8] Acidophils which secrete growth hormone, and in some species prolactin, contain granules about 350 mμ in diameter, which have been isolated and shown to contain G.H. activity. Similar cells with larger (400–700 mμ) and fewer granules have been shown in the rat and cow to contain prolactin, the cell-type for prolactin secretion in man has only recently been defined. Basophilic cells with granules of about 150 mμ diameter have been correlated with T.S.H. secretion, and those with somewhat larger granules (200 mμ) with gonadotrophin secretion. The normal A.C.T.H.-producing cells are probably also basophils, though some patients with Cushing's syndrome harbour chromophobe tumours. The granules in pituitary cells are storage forms of the protein hormones of the gland. Cells containing acidophilic granules predominate, and the pituitary contains much larger stores of G.H. than any other hormone.

The ultrastructure of protein-secreting exocrine and endocrine glands has been correlated with the biosynthetic activity of the secreting cells.[9] In gene transcription the information encoded in nuclear D.N.A. is read out as messenger R.N.A., which passes into the cytoplasm and becomes associated with several ribosomes to form polysomes. In protein-secreting cells the polysomes are found mainly on the outer surface of the intracellular cisternæ, producing the appearance of the rough endoplasmic reticulum. Here, aminoacids carried by transfer R.N.A. are assembled on the ribosomes, according to the order of codons (base triplets) in the messenger R.N.A. to form specific proteins. The growing protein chain is thought to enter the lumen of the endoplasmic reticulum, migrate to the Golgi region, and pass into the Golgi complex as vesicles of protein which coalesce to form granules enclosed by a membrane. During secretion, the

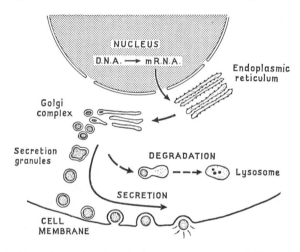

Fig. 4—Formation and release of secretory granules by a pituitary acidophil.
Modified from Fawcett et al.[9]

membrane of the granule fuses with the cell membrane, and the hormone is released as granules or molecules into the perivascular space (fig. 4).

In endocrine glands, the sequence of events is similar, although the endocrine cells have a lower secretion-rate. Stimulation of specific physiological activities is associated with increase in endoplasmic reticulum and enlargement of the Golgi complex in specific cell populations: for instance, during lactation in the rat and broodiness in the turkey these organelles are extremely prominent in the prolactin-producing cells. When the need for a stored hormone is reduced, lysosomes clear the cell of redundant secretion granules. There is good evidence that hormones are secreted from pituitary cells by membrane coalescence and granule extrusion. At high rates of hormone secretion and release, the cell product may not be concentrated into granules but be discharged from pallid vesicles with essentially fluid contents. This mechanism is consistent with the occurrence of hormonal hypersecretion by chromophobe tumours in patients with Cushing's syndrome and acromegaly, and by poorly granulated cells in animals after end-organ ablation.

Pituitary Hormones

The molecular weights of the peptide hormones A.C.T.H., M.S.H., and G.H. are known, but the molecular weights of the glycoprotein hormones (T.S.H., L.H., F.S.H.) are still uncertain because of a tendency for the subunits of these hormones to aggregate. The structure and sequence of the peptide hormones is also known, that of H.G.H. being described in 1966 and revised in 1970.[10] The structure of the glycoprotein hormones has been much more difficult to determine, owing to their much lower concentration in the pituitary and the difficulties presented by the carbohydrate moiety of the molecule. The total carbohydrate component of pituitary F.S.H. comprises about 27% of the weight of the protein, 7% being composed of sialic acid, which is essential for the biological activity of the molecule in vivo. The carbohydrate content of L.H. is lower, with only 2% sialic acid. The sialic-acid residues of gonadotrophins are necessary for normal metabolism of the molecules. In their absence, gonadotrophins retain intrinsic biological activity but are extremely rapidly cleared from the circulation and cannot activate their target tissues in vivo.

The figures for pituitary hormone storage and secretion, derived and calculated from a number of sources, are shown in table I. The specific activities of the most purified preparations are shown in terms of the arbitrary units which have been chosen for biological standardisation of the individual pituitary hormones. These values are not absolute but give a useful indication of the quantities of each hormone stored in the gland and secreted each day in normal circumstances. The large stores and high secretion-rate of H.G.H. are especially prominent and accentuate our relative ignorance of the functions of this hormone in adult life.

TABLE I—PITUITARY HORMONE SECRETION

Hormone	Molecular weight	Pituitary content (μg.)	Secretion-rate (μg. per day)	Plasma-level (ng. per ml.)	Metabolic clearance rate (litres per day)	Probable specific activity of pure hormone (units per mg.)
A.C.T.H.	4500	300	10	0·03	300	200
H.G.H.	21,500	8500	500	1·0–5·0	280	2
T.S.H.	26,000	300	110	1·0–2·0	61	30
L.H.	30,000	80	30	0·5–1·5	36	14,000
F.S.H.	41,000	35	15	0·5–1·0	19	14,000

Posterior-pituitary Function

The posterior pituitary secretes two octapeptides with molecular weights of about 1200. Vasopressin (antidiuretic hormone [A.D.H.]) conserves body-water by reducing water excretion by the kidney, while oxytocin affects lactation and uterine muscle contraction. These peptides are thought to be synthesised in the hypothalamus and transported along axons to the posterior pituitary, from which they are secreted into the circulation. The neurons of the supra-opticohypophyseal tract do not synapse with other neurons but terminate in blood-spaces in the posterior pituitary. Large stores of vasopressin and oxytocin are contained in small neurosecretory granules in these neurons, each granule consisting of a "packet" of hormone in non-covalent association with specific binding proteins known as neurophysin.[11] 10–20% of the vasopressin is ready for release into the circulation, together with neurophysin. Prolonged dehydration results in enlargement of the neurohypophysis and the disappearance of characteristic neurohypophyseal proteins from the electrophoretic pattern of gland extracts. A.D.H. is probably synthesised in the supraoptic nucleus, and oxytocin in the paraventricular nucleus.

The neurophypophyseal systems of various vertebrates have been found to contain seven defined octapeptides, with two types of biological activity. Vasopressor-antidiuretic activity is seen in arginine-vasopressin, lysine-vasopressin, and arginine-vasotocin, while oxytocic milk-ejection activity is seen in oxytocin and related peptides. The mammalian pituitary contains only oxytocin and arginine-vasopressin (except the pig, which contains lysine-vasopressin). The hybrid peptide, arginine-vasotocin, is the antidiuretic hormone in amphibia and was synthesised chemically before its discovery in the amphibian pituitary (fig. 5). In an evolutionary sense, vasotocin is

ARGININE VASOTOCIN
Developmentally oldest neurohypophyseal peptide

Cys-Tyr-**Ileu**-Glu(NH$_2$)-Asp(NH$_2$)-Cys-Pro-**Arg**-Gly(NH$_2$)

OXYTOCIN
Mammalian oxytocic and milk-ejection factor

Cys-Tyr-**Ileu**-Glu(NH$_2$)-Asp(NH$_2$)-Cys-Pro-**Leu**-Gly(NH$_2$)

ARGININE-VASOPRESSIN
Mammalian A.D.H.

Cys-Tyr-**Phe**-Glu(NH$_2$)-Asp(NH$_2$)-Cys-Pro-**Arg**-Gly(NH$_2$)

LYSINE-VASOPRESSIN
Swine A.D.H.

Cys-Tyr-**Phe**-Glu(NH$_2$)-Asp(NH$_2$)-Cys-Pro-**Lys**-Gly(NH$_2$)

Fig. 5—The major neurohypophyseal peptides.

believed to be the oldest peptide and is found in most vertebrate groups from cyclostomes to birds. The first development of separate oxytocic hormones occurred in cartilaginous fish. Lysine-vasopressin appears to be an aberrant form of arginine-vasopressin and is found only in the pig.

Antidiuretic Hormone

Secretion of A.D.H. is stimulated by dehydration, saline loading, exercise, and hæmorrhage and is inhibited by water-loading and alcohol intake. The cells of the supraoptic nucleus appear to respond directly to changes of plasma-osmolality and indirectly to changes in plasma-volume. A.D.H. secretion is increased by rising plasma-osmolality and falling plasma-volume, and decreased by the reverse changes.

A.D.H. is cleared rapidly from the circulation and stimulates adenyl-cyclase activity and resorption of water, sodium, and urea in renal-tubular cells. It may affect water transport directly through functional "pores" in the cell membrane, and indirectly through increased sodium and urea concentration in the renal medulla.

Disorders of A.D.H. secretion occur in diabetes insipidus, which is due to congenital or acquired lesions in the neurohypophyseal system. The nephrogenic form of diabetes insipidus, which is usually familial, is due to end-organ resistance to vasopressin. Excessive A.D.H. secretion occurs in some intracerebral disorders, notably tuberculous meningitis, and in some cases of lung cancer in which the tumour itself produces large quantities of A.D.H. Synthetic lysine-vasopressin is the most convenient and satisfactory form of therapy for A.D.H. deficiency.

Oxytocin

In mammals oxytocin stimulates myoepithelial cells of the mammary gland to cause milk ejection. The afferent stimulus in this neuro-endocrine reflex is suckling or conditioning factors related to suckling. In women oxytocin release stimulated by suckling causes uterine contraction, which can be inhibited by alcohol ingestion. In the œstrous cow oxytocin is released when the bull comes into sight, causing uterine contractions which become strongest during coitus and which may assist sperm transport. Although oxytocin is not thought to affect mammary development and milk formation in women, studies on self-licking in pregnant rats and milking stimuli in virgin goats suggest that nipple stimulation encourages the development of lobuloalveolar breast tissue. This effect is probably due to stimulation of anterior-pituitary hormones, particularly prolactin, in these species.

Oxytocin does not seem to be involved in the initiation of labour. Hypophysectomised women and monkeys can reach term and begin labour without oxytocin substitution therapy, as do patients with diabetes insipidus. In normal women, the blood-level of oxytocin does not rise until labour is advanced. The stimulatory effects of oxytocin on the uterus probably accelerate completion of delivery.[12]

1. Harris, G. W. Neural Control of the Pituitary Gland. London, 1955.
2. Martini, L., Ganong, W. F. Neuroendocrinology. New York, 1966.
3. Guillemin, R. A. Rev. Physiol. 1967, **29**, 313.
4. Schally, A. V., Arimura, A., Bowers, C. Y., Kastin, A. J., Sawano, S., Redding, T. W. Rec. Prog. Horm. Res. 1968, **24**, 497.
5. Bruce, H. M. in Effects of External Stimuli on Reproduction (edited by G. E. W. Wolstenholme and M. O'Connor); p. 29. Boston, 1967.

6. Wurtman, R. J., Anton-Tay, F. *Rec. Prog. Horm. Res.* 1969, **25**, 443.
7. Barraclough, C. A. *ibid.* 1966, **22**, 503.
8. McShan, W. H., Hartley, M. W. *Rev. Physiol. exp. Pharmac.* 1965, **56**, 264.
9. Fawcett, D. W., Long, J. A., Jones, A. L. *Rec. Prog. Horm. Res.* 1969. **25**, 315.
10. Li, C. H., Liu, W., Dixon, J. S. *J. Am. chem. Soc.* 1966, **88**, 2050.
11. Sachs, H., Fawcett, P., Takabatake, Y., Portanova, R. *Rec. Prog. Horm. Res.* 1969, **25**, 447.
12. Csapo, A. I., Wood, C. Recent Advances in Endocrinology (edited by J. James); p. 207. Boston, 1968.

CHAPTER THREE

Growth Hormone

THE importance of the pituitary gland in growth regulation was recognised by Hutchinson, who proposed in 1900 that disturbances of pituitary function would result in dwarfism, gigantism, or acromegaly. The association of acromegaly with a pituitary lesion had been known since 1887, but the abnormality had not been identified as glandular oversecretion. Early studies on animals showed that hypophysectomy was followed by growth failure and gonadal atrophy, and by 1912 the concept of pituitary hypersecretion as the cause of acromegaly was accepted by Cushing, who referred to the "hormone of growth" in his book on the pituitary and its disorders. The existence of a pituitary growth factor was conclusively demonstrated by Evans in 1921, when anterior pituitary extracts were shown to produce gigantism in rats. Pituitary extracts were later shown to restore the growth-rate of hypophysectomised animals, and to produce a condition resembling acromegaly in dogs.

The restoration of body growth in hypophysectomised rats was developed into a specific bioassay for G.H. activity and used to monitor the purification of G.H. from pituitary extracts, culminating in the purification of bovine G.H. in 1944. Further studies on the effects of purified G.H. upon hypophysectomised and intact animals have given much information about the actions of G.H. on cell growth and metabolism. However, the physiological control mechanisms for H.G.H. secretion have not been clarified, despite the development of methods for measurement of the hormone in blood.

Actions of Growth Hormone

The long-term actions of G.H. on body growth are based upon numerous more acute effects on cellular activity and metabolism, particularly in muscle, adipose tissue, cartilage, and other connective tissues. These actions have been demonstrated by studies on the effects of hypophysectomy, replacement therapy with G.H., and excess G.H. administration to intact normal animals. Hypophysectomy severely reduces biosynthetic activities in many tissues and impairs carbohydrate metabolism. D.N.A. replication ceases in liver and muscle of growing animals, with loss rather than the usual increase of muscle cells with age.[1] Thymidine incorporation into D.N.A. of cartilage and adipose tissue is also diminished, and synthesis of liver R.N.A. is reduced. In connective tissue, synthesis of mucopolysaccharides and collagen is diminished, with reduced sulphate incorporation and hydroxyproline excretion. The low fasting blood-sugar and liver-glycogen levels of hypophysectomised animals are mainly due to the accompanying adrenal insufficiency and can be corrected by glucocorticoid administration. Two specific effects of G.H. deficiency on carbohydrate metabolism are decreased insulin secretion in response to a glucose load and increased sensitivity to exogenous insulin, with delayed recovery from insulin-induced hypoglycæmia.

The effects of G.H. in hypophysectomised animals include renewed D.N.A. replication and R.N.A. synthesis in liver, muscle, adipose tissue, and cartilage. Body growth is resumed, with increase in muscle mass and decrease in body fat. Nitrogen retention is pronounced, insulin secretion and insulin tolerance are restored to normal, sulphur-35 incorporation into cartilage and skin mucopolysaccharide is stimulated, and hydroxyproline excretion is raised, reflecting increased collagen synthesis and turnover. Stimulation of cartilage formation in hypophysectomised animals is the basis of the tibial-epiphyseal-line bioassay for G.H. activity. Normal endochondral osteogenesis requires both G.H. and an adequate level of thyroxine secretion.

As well as these effects on specific tissues, G.H. also influences the intermediary metabolism of protein, carbohydrate, and lipids. The blood-levels of urea and aminoacids are lowered, reflecting the reduced catabolism and enhanced cellular uptake of aminoacids for protein synthesis in muscle, liver, adipose tissue, and other connective tissues. Mobilisation of fat from adipose tissue is stimulated, and plasma-free-fatty-acids are elevated. The effects on carbohydrate metabolism are more complex—an early fall of blood-sugar and free fatty acids after H.G.H. injection reflects an insulin-like effect, in contrast to the later effects of enhanced gluconeogenesis, fat mobilisation, and impaired carbohydrate tolerance which are seen in varying degrees in different species. In addition, G.H. increases the plasma-insulin reponse to glucose, though the basal secretion of insulin is only slightly elevated.

In dogs and cats, large doses of G.H. can cause hyperglycæmia and diabetes mellitus. The diabetogenic action of G.H. in the dog is due largely to an inhibitory effect of G.H. on glucose uptake by tissues and not to exhaustion of insulin secretion. Similar effects can be seen in other species after islet-cell activity is reduced. In man, large doses of G.H. are normally needed to produce diabetogenic effects, but in patients with impaired pancreatic reserve such effects can be induced with much smaller quantities. This is most obvious in hypophysectomised diabetic patients, in whom quite small doses of H.G.H. (1 mg.) can produce striking hyperglycæmia and ketosis.[2] Thus, the diabetogenic action of G.H. may not be apparent in the presence of adequate insulin secretion but is revealed when islet-cell function is reduced. The antagonism of peripheral insulin action by G.H. has been clearly shown in man during study of glucose utilisation by forearm muscle. H.G.H. blocks the insulin-induced uptake of glucose by muscle without affecting the action of insulin on free-fatty-acid release.[3]

The other effects of H.G.H. in man include nitrogen retention, reduced blood-urea, increased plasma-free-fatty-acids, and retention of Na^+, Cl^-, K^+, Mg^{++}, and Ca^{++}, the last despite increased urinary excretion of Ca^{++}. When administered to other species, H.G.H. shows several prolactin-like properties. These include mammogenic and lactogenic actions in rodents and rabbits, stimulation of the pigeon crop sac, and luteotrophic action on the rodent ovary. This prolactin-like activity associated with the H.G.H. molecule is not present in the G.H. molecules of those species which possess a separate prolactin molecule. H.G.H. has been shown to increase lactation in women, but most attempts to detect increased G.H. secretion during lactation have been negative. Lactation can occur in women with isolated H.G.H. deficiency, so that H.G.H. secretion seems not to be essential for lactation.

Species Specificity of Growth Hormone

Since the isolation of bovine G.H. in 1944,[4] purified preparations of G.H. have been isolated from pituitary extracts of man, monkey, sheep, whale, pig, horse, and rat. Although bovine, human, and many other varieties of growth hormone are active in the rat, only primate G.H. is effective in man. Species specificity in the biological activity of growth hormone is due to physicochemical variations in molecular structure; whereas animals such as the rat respond to G.H. from many species, primates cannot respond to the active sites of G.H. molecules from other species. Preparations of human and monkey G.H. stimulate growth in man and other species, and the primary structure of H.G.H. has been determined. The hormone is a single polypeptide chain of 188 aminoacid residues, with a molecular weight of 21,500. The molecule can survive partial degradation by enzymes without loss of biological activity, as well as a degree of chemical modification.[5] Although similarities of structure are detectable in bovine G.H. by sequence analysis, and in a variety of nonprimate growth hormones by complement fixation, human tissues cannot recognise these similarities and will respond only to primate G.H. An active "common core" in the G.H. molecules of all species has been postulated, and biological activity of enzyme-treated bovine G.H. in man has been described. However, such preparations are difficult to achieve in a reproducible fashion and are of variable biological activity and highly antigenic when administered to human subjects.

Secretion of Growth Hormone

The pituitary content of H.G.H. is remarkably high—5-15 mg. per gland, compared with microgramme quantities of L.H., F.S.H., and T.S.H. In most species G.H. is visible as a prominent band on electrophoresis of saline extracts of pituitary tissue. The hormone is relatively robust, and H.G.H. can be prepared in good yield from frozen and acetone-dried glands, and even from embalmed glands. Combined extracts of G.H., F.S.H., T.S.H., and A.C.T.H. can be prepared by several isolation techniques. The daily production-rate of H.G.H. is about 500 μg., and secretion continues from childhood until old age. Secretion of G.H. has been extensively studied in several species by radioimmunoassay of plasma-G.H. levels, yet the role of the hormone in adult life has not been completely elucidated. Plasma-levels of H.G.H. vary considerably in normal subjects, according to age, sex, activity, stress, and metabolic factors. In the newborn, H.G.H. levels are extremely high, especially during the first few weeks of life, even though G.H. does not seem to be essential for fetal and neonatal growth. Thereafter, the basal level of H.G.H. is 1-5 ng. per ml. in normal subjects, with intermittent pulses of secretion which may raise plasma-H.G.H. to 25 ng. per ml. or more. These spikes of plasma-G.H. occur most often after activity, during deep sleep, especially in children, and several hours after meals. Such peaks are commoner in women, occurring most frequently midway through the menstrual cycle and during œstrogen administration. The greater secretory capacity of the female is accompanied by increased responsiveness to certain stimuli, such as exercise and arginine infusion. These intermittent peaks of plasma-G.H. level occasionally complicate the assessment of pituitary function by G.H. assay but can be readily distinguished from pathological elevations by their ready suppression after glucose administration.

The secretion of G.H. by pituitary acidophils is regulated by the G.H.-releasing hormone of the hypothalamus (G.H.R.F.). This factor is demonstrable in crude hypothalamic extracts, but there is some doubt about the ability of purified extracts to cause G.H. release as detected by radioimmunoassay, whereas bioassay studies in rodents showed considerable activity in such preparations. G.H.R.F. has been isolated and identified as a small acidic peptide of 11 aminoacid residues. The hypothalamic content of G.H.R.F. is reduced in animals by starvation and corticosteroid treatment, and is increased by thyroxine. The importance of thyroxine for G.H. secretion is well known in the rat, since thyroidectomy leads to striking reduction of G.H. synthesis and storage in this species.

G.H. synthesis and storage as characteristic granules in pituitary acidophilic cells of well-defined histological and electron-microscopical appearance has been demonstrated in several species. In rodents, ruminants, and birds somewhat similar cells with larger granules have been shown to produce prolactin, but the evidence for prolactin formation in man has until recently been less conclusive. The presence of prolactin activity in H.G.H. preparations and the difficulty of detecting prolactin in man led to speculation that both activities reside in the same molecule in primates. Observations on prolactin secreting pituitary tumours, plasma-prolactin levels bioassayed during lactation, and the presence of prolactin-secreting cells in the human pituitary during pregnancy supported the existence of a separate prolactin molecule in man, and specific radioimmunoassays have shown high plasma-prolactin levels during pregnancy and lactation.

Although the identification of human prolactin proved difficult, an analogous hormone is formed in large quantities by the primate placenta. This protein was described in 1962 by Josimovich and MacLaren[6] and termed human placental lactogen (H.P.L.) because of its lactogenic activity on the pigeon crop and rabbit mammary gland. It has substantial structural and immunological similarities to H.G.H. and shows weak G.H. activity. By analogy with human chorionic gonadotrophin (H.C.G.), it is also called human chorionic somatomammotrophin (H.C.S.). So far, the function of H.C.S. has not been determined, but obviously it does not function as a prolactin in the usual sense, because it is not secreted after delivery. The large quantities of H.C.S. secreted in pregnancy seem to suppress H.G.H. release and stimulate mammary development, though not to the lactation stage. It is possible that the sudden termination of H.C.S. secretion at delivery is involved in the initiation of lactation. Although the growth activity of H.C.S. is extremely slight in man, the quantites secreted during pregnancy reach 1–2 g. daily near term, with blood-levels of 5–10 μg. per ml. These large amounts of H.C.S. could account for many of the metabolic changes of pregnancy, especially raised plasma-free-fatty-acid levels and lowered peripheral glucose uptake by tissues, and are probably responsible for the exacerbation of diabetes mellitus during pregnancy.

H.C.S. secretion rises steadily during normal pregnancy, in contrast to the early rise and subsequent fall of H.C.G. secretion by the placenta. The origin and short half-life of H.C.S. make it a relatively sensitive indication of trophoblastic function and mass, and the blood-level of H.C.S. has been shown to fall some days before spontaneous abortion. It has also been proposed that blood-levels of H.C.S. may be used to assess risk to the fetoplacental unit, and that frequent estimations in high-risk patients will complement the results of urinary œstriol determinations.

Factors Affecting Growth-hormone Secretion[7]

Measurement of plasma-H.G.H. can only be done by radioimmunossay, using antiserum to H.G.H. and radioiodinated G.H. tracer to establish the saturation-analysis system. The studies of Roth et al.[8] first revealed the lability of G.H. secretion and its relation to metabolic and stressful stimuli. Radioimmunossays for estimation of plasma-G.H. in monkey, sheep, cow, dog, rabbit, and rat have also been developed. These sometimes produce results which conflict with those obtained by bioassay of pituitary G.H. content and with the pattern of G.H. response which is seen in man; such differences emphasise the importance of interpreting the results of G.H. radioimmunoassay with caution. The levels of immunoreactive growth hormone in plasma have never been adequately correlated with biological activity except in conditions of G.H. hypersecretion, such as acromegaly.

Insulin-induced Hypoglycæmia

This is the most consistent stimulus to H.G.H. secretion; to be effective, blood-sugar should fall to 50% or less of the basal level. Smaller falls of blood-glucose are much less consistently effective, and it is unlikely that physiological fluctuations in blood-glucose could constitute a stimulus to G.H. secretion. Apart from acutely induced absolute hypoglycæmia, decreases of blood-sugar from a previously high level can also provoke G.H. release, as can further falls of blood-sugar in patients with chronic hypoglycæmia. Interference with intracellular glucose utilisation by administration of 2-deoxyglucose will also stimulate G.H. secretion in man. Conversely, administration of glucose causes an initial suppression of H.G.H. secretion, followed by a rise after 3–4 hours.

Fasting

Starvation causes a rise in plasma-G.H. in man, rat, and rabbit, though not in sheep. This has been interpreted as a sign of the role of G.H. as a hormone of fasting, increasing fat mobilisation and slowing down glucose utilisation. However, the response to fasting in man is rather variable, and it is not proven that G.H. plays a major role in metabolic homœostasis in fasting. It may influence basal levels of lipolysis and the insulin response to glucose, but much of the metabolic adaptation to fasting seems to depend on decreased insulin secretion and the ratio of insulin to G.H. in plasma, rather than upon the absolute level of G.H.

In severe malnutrition plasma-G.H. levels are sometimes very high. In children with marasmus and kwashiorkor Pimstone et al.[9] found consistently high plasma-G.H. levels, which could be returned to normal by protein feeding. The elevation of plasma-G.H. in these children could not be correlated with such parameters as serum-albumin level but seemed directly related to protein intake. Analogous hypersecretion of H.G.H. has also been observed in disorders associated with less severe degrees of malnutrition, such as anorexia nervosa and mucoviscidosis.

Exercise

Plasma-levels of H.G.H. may rise after quite light activity, the elevation showing some correlation with the severity of exercise. The rise is usually transient, levels returning to baseline despite continued activity. The most striking responses are seen in subjects who are physically unfit and may be related to the degree of lactate production.

Aminoacid Infusion

The demonstration that protein ingestion and aminoacid infusion caused insulin secretion led to the speculation that the release of G.H. may be similarly stimulated, causing a concerted action of the two hormones on blood-glucose level and protein synthesis. Infusion of aminoacids in high concentration provokes growth-hormone secretion in the female, leading to raised plasma-H.G.H. levels comparable with those occurring after insulin hypoglycæmia. This response also occurs erratically in males, though œstrogen treatment will enhance the magnitude and frequency of response.[10] Some workers have reported equal responses in males and females, but this variation may be related to the preparation of the patients for study, for ambulation and activity before testing could produce misleadingly high G.H. levels. The elicitation of a specific arginine response to H.G.H. is best seen in the fasting rested female subject. Although the response may be obscured by fluctuations related to activity, spontaneous or induced H.G.H. peaks during testing provide a useful index of normal pituitary function. These responses to arginine do not necessarily indicate a physiological relation between aminoacid level and H.G.H. secretion, since rather high levels are needed for stimulation, and the effect is largely confined to the female. Protein meals also produce a rise in plasma-H.G.H., again most consistently in the female.

Stress

Various forms of stress, such as surgery, emotional stress, bacterial endotoxins, and vasopressin stimulate H.G.H. secretion. Other stimuli, such as insulin hypoglycæmia, may also operate through a stress mechanism, possibly involving the actions of catecholamines and A.C.T.H.

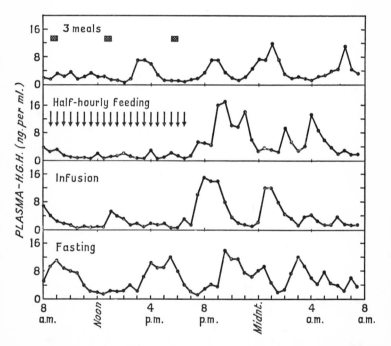

Fig. 6—Patterns of H.G.H. secretion in a normal subject under various metabolic conditions: (i) 3 meals daily; (ii) half-hourly feeding; (iii) continuous intravenous infusion of glucose; and (iv) fasting.

Levels were highest during fasting and were suppressed by frequent feeding, but not for more than four hours by continuous glucose infusion. The nocturnal peaks of secretion are apparent during each study. (After Glick and Goldsmith.[11])

Neural Stimuli

As well as the neurogenic component of stress-induced H.G.H. release, there are other neural stimuli which increase H.G.H. secretion—e.g., anticipation of unpleasant sensations (such as symptomatic insulin hypoglycæmia), fear, and noise. Large peaks of H.G.H. often occur at the onset of deep sleep. The intermittent spikes of H.G.H. secretion in normal subjects are suppressed for only a short time by continuous glucose administration, further spikes appearing after a few hours despite continued or increased glucose intake (fig. 6).[11] The periodic bursts of H.G.H. secretion in normal subjects seem to be triggered by a central-nervous-system mechanism responding to stressful and exaggerated metabolic stimuli but not apparently related to any measurable physiological variables involved in G.H. secretion. The large spikes of plasma-G.H. must reflect the simultaneous release of numerous secretory granules from the acidophils in response to stimuli from the hypothalamus.

An extreme example of cerebral effects on H.G.H. secretion is seen in severely emotionally deprived children, in whom growth retardation is sometimes associated with decreased G.H. secretion.[12] This is part of a syndrome of temporary hypopituitarism, and is reversed by removal from the adverse environment.

Effects of Hormones on Growth-hormone Secretion

Thyroid Hormone

Hypothyroidism is associated with decreased synthesis, storage, and release of growth hormone, and with growth retardation. The G.H. content of the rat pituitary is greatly reduced after thyroidectomy, and, in man, the H.G.H. response to stimuli is reduced in hypothyroidism. The growth-rate is restored to normal by thyroid replacement before the H.G.H. response becomes normal, because thyroid hormone has a direct effect upon growth in addition to its synergistic action on growth-hormone secretion. The production-rate of growth hormone is much lower than normal in hypothyroidism and is higher than normal in hyperthyroidism.

Sex Hormones

Œstrogens strongly influence both G.H. synthesis and the G.H. secretory response to stimuli. They inhibit G.H. secretion in the rat, but stimulate it in human beings. Women have higher basal levels of H.G.H. and more frequent pulses of H.G.H. secretion than men. They also show enhanced responsiveness to stimuli such as activity and arginine infusion, which is most apparent midway through the menstrual cycle and during œstrogen administration.[13] In men, œstrogen treatment also leads to enhancement of the plasma-H.G.H. response to arginine infusion. Androgen treatment stimulates G.H. secretion in the rat and may increase G.H. responsiveness in man. High doses of progestagens can suppress the H.G.H. response to insulin hypoglycæmia.

Corticosteroids and A.C.T.H.

The effects of corticosteroid therapy on G.H. secretion vary according to the dosage and duration of treatment. In general, corticosteroids inhibit the G.H. response, especially to insulin hypoglycæmia. Patients with Cushing's syndrome are often unresponsive to hypoglycæmia, whereas addisonian patients show increased G.H. responses to insulin hypoglycæmia and other stimuli.

In contrast to the action of corticosteroids, A.C.T.H. infusion can stimulate H.G.H. release and responsiveness to insulin hypoglycæmia. The release of A.C.T.H. and catecholamines may be part of the sequence of events leading to H.G.H. release in response to stressful stimuli.

Catecholamines

Infusion of small doses of adrenaline does not provoke H.G.H. release in man, though larger doses cause elevation of plasma-G.H., as may cyclic A.M.P. infusion. The effects of adrenergic blockade on the H.G.H. response to insulin hypoglycæmia indicate that α-adrenergic receptors enhance G.H. secretion, while β-receptors have an inhibitory effect. This is the opposite of the pattern of adrenergic control of insulin secretion. It has been suggested that A.C.T.H. and catecholamines may stimulate H.G.H. secretion and lipid mobilisation during fasting, whereas insulin secretion is inhibited by catecholamines and antagonised peripherally by H.G.H.

Growth-hormone Secretion in Man

Assessment of the ability of the pituitary to secrete H.G.H. provides specific information in patients with growth disorders and acromegaly: it is also an index of pituitary function in suspected hypopituitarism. The most widely used stimulus to H.G.H. secretion is insulin-induced hypoglycæmia, with a fall of blood-sugar to 50% or less of the basal level and preferably mild clinical manifestations of hypoglycæmia (fig. 7).

0·1–0·15 units of insulin per kg. of body-weight is injected intravenously. Blood-samples are taken for glucose, H.G.H., and cortisol determination before, and at intervals for 2 hours after, the injection. In normal subjects, a satisfactory fall in blood-sugar is usually seen after 20–30 minutes, and a sharp rise in plasma-H.G.H. occurs 30–90 minutes after insulin. This test does not give false positive results, since any rise in H.G.H. secretion suggests relatively normal pituitary function. (A.C.T.H. release can also be detected with this test by following the plasma-cortisol response.[14]) If a negative H.G.H. response is obtained the test should be repeated, or followed by an alternative standard stimulus, before impaired H.G.H. secretion is diagnosed.

The other commonly used stimulus to H.G.H. release is intravenous infusion of aminoacids in high concentration—usually 30 g. arginine

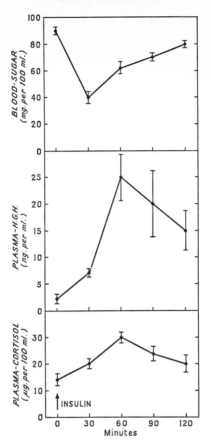

Fig. 7—Effect of insulin-induced hypoglycæmia on plasma-H.G.H. in 6 normal subjects (mean ± S.E.M.).

In most subjects the rise in H.G.H. secretion is accompanied by an elevation of plasma-cortisol. Thus, the insulin-hypoglycæmia test provides information about the secretion of both H.G.H. and A.C.T.H. by the pituitary. In patients with growth-hormone deficiency, no rise in plasma-H.G.H. occurs, and the return of blood-sugar to normal levels is somewhat delayed. In hypopituitarism these features are often accompanied by absent plasma-cortisol response to hypoglycæmia.

monohydrochloride in distilled water over a period of 30 minutes— resulting, in women, in a rise of plasma-H.G.H. comparable to that caused by insulin hypoglycæmia, but often a much smaller rise in men. (The relative responses of men and women has differed considerably in various studies, possibly because specific responses to arginine have been obscured by spontaneous H.G.H. peaks in subjects who have been active and ambulatory before testing.) The usual order for pituitary-function testing by evaluation of H.G.H. secretion is insulin hypoglycæmia, followed by arginine infusion if no H.G.H. response is elicited by hypoglycæmia. Other stimuli which have been used to provoke H.G.H. release include 2-deoxyglucose, pyromen, glucagon, and lysine-vasopressin, while A.C.T.H. infusion may provide a further useful stimulus.

Suppressibility of H.G.H. secretion during diagnostic testing can be examined by oral or intravenous administration of glucose. Usually, 50 g. glucose is given by mouth, and blood-glucose and plasma-H.G.H. levels are measured during the next 2 hours. The plasma-G.H. level is initially reduced, then rises again a few hours later. Although continuous glucose loading cannot maintain this inhibition of G.H. secretion, the acute response is extremely constant in normal subjects. This sensitivity to glucose is not present in the newborn but develops several weeks after birth. Absence of suppression in the adult is seen most often in acromegaly, and glucose loading is essential to confirm this diagnosis in acromegalic patients with low or moderate plasma-H.G.H. levels (fig. 8).

As well as these two clearcut effects of glucose loading on G.H. secretion in normal and acromegalic subjects, a third response to glucose is seen in some disorders. This is a "paradoxical elevation" of plasma-H.G.H. soon after glucose ingestion, instead of the usual suppression. This response has been seen in premature infants, children with hypothalamic lesions, some acromegalic patients with low basal H.G.H. levels, and in patients with cerebral tumour, acute intermittent porphyria, prediabetes, Turner's syndrome, myocardial infarction, uræmia, chronic active hepatitis, and some cases of lung cancer. Although there is no outstanding common feature in these diverse conditions, all appear to be associated with an abnormality of glucose feedback upon the central-nervous-system-controlled pulsatile secretion of G.H., leading to abolition of the early suppressing effect of glucose and advancement or enhancement of the later stimulation of H.G.H. secretion.

In hypopituitarism, basal levels of H.G.H. are low or normal, but do not respond to insulin-induced hypoglycæmia or arginine infusion. In acromegaly, plasma-H.G.H. levels are usually very high (20–250 ng. per ml.) and unresponsive to glucose suppression. In a few acromegalic patients plasma-H.G.H. levels are in the upper normal range but are not suppressed by glucose, which sometimes evokes para-

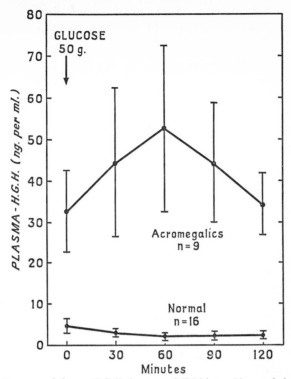

Fig. 8—Response of plasma-H.G.H. (mean ± S.E.M.) to a 50 g. oral glucose load in normal subjects and acromegalic patients.

H.G.H. levels are suppressed in normal subjects but not in acromegalics. In some acromegalics, partial suppression may occur; in others, paradoxical rises of H.G.H. levels are sometimes seen.

doxical hypersecretion of H.G.H. Despite these occasional paradoxical responses, a clear indication of the state of H.G.H. secretion can usually be obtained by the response to insulin hypoglycæmia, followed when necessary by arginine infusion and glucose suppression.

Fluctuation of H.G.H. secretion makes the estimation of secretion-rates difficult. Urinary excretion of H.G.H. is not a useful index of secretion, for the amount excreted is very low and is not proportional to the endogenous secretion-rate. Estimations of secretion-rate have been obtained by measuring the metabolic clearance-rate of labelled H.G.H.— i.e., the volume of blood cleared of H.G.H., in litres per day. This value, multiplied by the peripheral-blood level of H.G.H. in microgrammes per litre, gives the secretion-rate in microgrammes per day. This is about 500 μg. per day in men, and somewhat higher in women. Low secretion-rates have been observed in diabetes and hypothyroidism, and decreased metabolism of H.G.H. has been seen in patients with renal failure and hepatic failure.

Disorders of Growth-hormone Secretion (fig. 9)

Hypopituitary Dwarfism

Dwarfism in children with organic lesions adjacent to the pituitary is an obvious consequence of G.H. deficiency, resulting either from

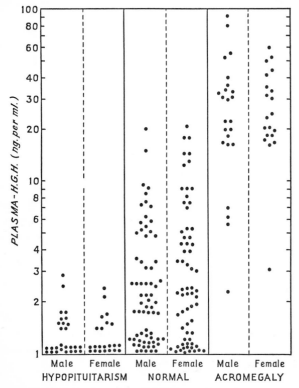

Fig. 9—Basal H.G.H. levels in normal subjects and in patients with hypopituitarism and acromegaly.

There is considerable overlap between hypopituitarism and normal levels; insulin-induced hypoglycæmia, arginine infusion, and vasopressin administration stimulate the normal pituitary to secrete growth hormone and are used to distinguish between low normal and hypopituitary levels of plasma-H.G.H. There is much less overlap between acromegalic and normal values, and the response to glucose suppression can be used to distinguish high normal from low acromegalic results.

the primary lesion or from surgical treatment. Idiopathic hypopituitarism can also cause dwarfism, as can isolated deficiency of H.G.H. secretion. The association of growth retardation with emotional deprivation and parental neglect is due to reversible hypopituitarism with defective A.C.T.H. and G.H. secretion. G.H. secretion and growthrate return to normal after removal from the adverse environment.

Hypopituitarism in childhood was often difficult to diagnose by indirect tests of pituitary function, but both diagnosis and treatment were made possible when purified H.G.H. became available. G.H. secretion in dwarfed children can be assessed by radioimmunoassay of plasma-H.G.H. and by plasma-G.H. responses to insulin hypoglycæmia and arginine infusion. Clinical features can sometimes give an indication of the disorder. Normal birth-weight, severe growth retardation, a tendency to obesity, and a low fasting blood-sugar with a delayed recovery from insulin hypoglycæmia are often seen in children with G.H. deficiency. After demonstration of absent G.H. secretion, the acute effect of H.G.H. administration on blood-urea, plasma-free-fatty-acids, and nitrogen retention can be determined, the last showing the best correlation with the long-term response of body growth.

In the majority of dwarfed children, including those with constitutional short stature, achondroplasia, gonadal dysgenesis, and other defects, H.G.H. secretion is normal and treatment with H.G.H. is ineffective. By contrast, the growth response of children with hypopituitarism and isolated G.H. deficiency is dramatic.

Growth hormone from the pituitaries of animals such as sheep and cows is inactive in man. Attempts to utilise these abundant sources of G.H. by chemical or enzymatic modifications of the G.H. molecule have been made in the hope of uncovering the active sequences. Structural analysis has revealed some similarity between bovine and human growth hormone, and bovine G.H. modified by controlled treatment with trypsin has produced acute metabolic effects in man.[15] Unfortunately, these preparations are highly antigenic when administered to children and evoke the appearance of antibodies which in some cases have shown cross-reaction with H.G.H.

H.C.S. (or H.P.L.) has been thought to be potentially useful in the treatment of pituitary dwarfism, since it is easily prepared from placentas and does not provoke antibody formation. However, the treatment of hypopituitary dwarfs with H.C.S. has not been followed by consistent growth effects, and various modifications of the native protein have also been inactive. Now that the primary structure of H.G.H. is known, it is likely that synthetic fragments of the molecule with growth activity will be prepared, analogous to the active sequences of A.C.T.H. and gastrin. It is also possible that a partial synthesis of growth-active peptides could be achieved by modification of fragments derived from H.C.S. or bovine G.H.

Isolated H.G.H. Deficiency

This may occur sporadically, or within families.[16] The pattern of inheritance of the familial form is that of an autosomal recessive gene. Affected patients show normal birth-weight, severe growth retardation in infancy, and no growth-hormone response to insulin-induced hypoglycæmia. Because normal sexual maturation can occur in patients with isolated G.H. deficiency, it is important to give treatment with H.G.H. before puberty, so that a growth response can be obtained before epiphyseal fusion occurs.

Secretion of Inactive H.G.H.

The possibility of this abnormality has been raised by the description of a family of children with elevated H.G.H. levels but severe growth retardation. This combination could be attributed to a pituitary abnormality resulting in the synthesis of H.G.H. molecules with normal immunological reactivity but abnormal in a critical sequence concerned with metabolic activity—a situation comparable to the abnormal hæmoglobins. This possibility is consistent with the observation that these dwarfs responded to treatment with exogenous H.G.H.

Lack of End-organ Response to Endogenous H.G.H.

African pygmies have some features which suggest H.G.H. deficiency—notably, pronounced growth retardation, unusually severe hypoglycæmia after standard doses of insulin, and a blunted plasma-insulin response to arginine infusion. However, the levels of plasma-H.G.H. rise in a normal way after hypoglycæmia and arginine infusion, so that G.H. release seems to be normal. That the pygmy's short stature is due to tissue unresponsiveness to H.G.H. rather than to the secretion of a functionally inactive H.G.H. molecule was suggested by examination of the metabolic effects of administered H.G.H. Long-term effects of H.G.H. have not been investigated in the pygmy, but the lack of effect of short-term treatment on plasma-free-fatty-acids, blood-urea, and the plasma-insulin responses to glucose and arginine probably indicate end-organ unresponsiveness to human growth hormone.[17]

Growth without Growth Hormone

Growth in the fetal and neonatal period is probably largely independent of growth-hormone secretion. Indeed, a normal birth-weight is usual in children with short stature due to deficient G.H. secretion, whereas low birth-weight is more characteristic of dwarfs in whom G.H. secretion is normal. In general, the dependence of later growth on normal G.H. secretion in unquestionable, but there are two situations in which growth seems out of proportion to the measured rate of H.G.H. secretion. The first is the "catch-up" growth seen in some children after several years of growth retardation caused by organic lesions of the hypothalamus and pituitary The other is cerebral gigantism, in which children are born large and remain large during development yet show normal G.H. secretion. In both these conditions, a permissive effect of minimal G.H. levels for normal growth and of normal G.H. levels for excessive growth could be invoked. However, these and other observations on G.H. levels under various conditions of growth and metabolism lead also to the speculation that the active circulating growth principle may not be identical to the immunoreactive G.H. measured in the plasma by radioimmunoassay.

One circulating factor which is evoked by G.H. and which has an effect upon cartilage metabolism has already been defined. This plasma "sulphation factor" is G.H.-dependent, stimulates sulphur-35 incorporation into cartilage, and is present in low concentrations in hypopituitarism and in high concentrations in acromegaly.[18] In addition, peptides with lipotrophic activity and effects upon carbohydrate metabolism have been prepared from G.H. by other investigators. These observations, together with the relative inactivity of G.H. on tissues in vitro and the difficulty of relating G.H. secretion to specific metabolic stimuli, suggest that pituitary G.H. may function as a precursor of the metabolically active peptides responsible for growth. Such derivatives may be released from the pituitary with varying quantities of the parent hormone, or they may be formed in peripheral tissues. There is increasing evidence that renal uptake and metabolism of G.H. may be an essential step in biological activation of the pituitary hormone, possibly by the formation of secondary peptides with growth and metabolic activity. The level of immunoreactive G.H. in blood may therefore relate only approximately to the production-rate of metabolically active growth-hormone, yet it can provide a useful index of overall pituitary function and acidophil-cell activity.

Acromegaly

The features of acromegaly are due entirely to the hypersecretion of H.G.H. and the local effects of the pituitary lesion. The pituitary tumours of acromegalic patients are commonly of chromophobe or mixed histological appearance, in accordance with their low storage and rapid secretion of G.H. Some cases of acromegaly may result from a primary hypothalamic disorder, with excessive secretion of G.H.R.F. leading to acidophil hyperplasia and ultimately to pituitary tumour. The majority of acromegalic patients have plasma-H.G.H. levels far above normal—20–200 ng. per ml. In addition, the serum of acromegalic patients has been shown to contain growth-active peptides which are distinct from growth hormone, and occasional patients have plasma-immunoreactive-H.G.H. levels within the normal range.

Most patients with active acromegaly require early treatment for both tumour growth and the effects of G.H. hypersecretion. When visual disturbance and other evidence of extrasellar spread is present, surgical resection is necessary. In many patients the tumour is confined to the pituitary fossa, and alternative ablation procedures have been devised. Conventional irradiation is ineffective, but proton-beam therapy has been moderately effective for the control of acromegaly and is probably the procedure of choice as an alternative to surgery. The method is atraumatic and has few serious complications; but it is not widely available, does not always achieve adequate G.H. suppression, and may require up to 2 years for full evaluation of the therapeutic effect.

Local irradiation has been performed by the trans-sphenoidal implantation of isotopes such as yttrium-90, but the technique has a fairly high frequency of infection and cerebrospinal-fluid rhinorrhœa. Cryogenic ablation of the pituitary has also been performed via the trans-sphenoidal route. All such procedures have the advantages of convenience and cosmetic effects but have a moderate frequency of complications and inadequate ablations. The further development of trans-sphenoidal surgical resection may prove to be the most satisfactory method of treatment.

1. Cheek, D. B. Human Growth: Body Composition, Cell Growth, Energy and Intelligence; p. 306. Philadelphia, 1968.
2. Ikkos, D., Luft, R. *Acta endocr., Copenh.* 1962, **39**, 567.
3. Zierler, K. L. *in* Clinical Endocrinology (edited by E. B. Astwood and C. E. Cassidy); vol. II, p. 55. Amsterdam, 1968.
4. Li, C. H., Evans, H. M. *Science, N.Y.* 1944, **99**, 183.
5. Li, C. H. *in* Growth Hormone (edited by A. Pecile and E. Muller); p. 3. Amsterdam, 1968.
6. Josimovich, J. B., MacLaren, J. A. *Endocrinology*, 1962, **71**, 209.
7. Glick, S. M. *in* Frontiers in Neuroendocrinology (edited by W. F. Ganong and L. Martini). London, 1969.
8. Roth, J., Glick, S. M., Yalow, R. S., Berson, S. A. *Metabolism*, 1963, **12**, 577.
9. Pimstone, B. L., Wittman, W., Hansen, J. D. L., Murray, P. *Am. J. clin. Nutr.* 1968, **21**, 482.
10. Rabinowitz, D., Merimee, T. J., Nelson, J. K., Schultz, R. B., Burgess, J. A. *in* Growth Hormone (edited by A. Pecile and E. Muller); p. 105. Amsterdam, 1968.
11. Glick, S. M., Goldsmith, S. *ibid.* p. 84.
12. Powell, G. F., Brasel, J. A., Raiti, S., Blizzard, R. M. *New Engl. J. Med.* 1967, **276**, 1279.
13. Frantz, A. G., Rabkin, M. T. *J. clin. Endocr.* 1965, **25**, 1470.
14. Landon, J., Greenwood, F. C., Stamp, T. C. B., Wynn, V. *J. clin. Invest.* 1966, **45**, 437.
15. Nadler, A. C., Sonenberg, M., New, M. I., Free, C. A. *Metabolism*, 1967, **16**, 830.
16. Rimoin, D. L., Merimee, T. J., Rabinowitz, D., Cavalli-Sforza, L. L., McKusick, V. A. *in* Growth Hormone (edited by A. Pecile and E. Muller); p. 418. Amsterdam, 1968.
17. Merimee, T. J., Rimoin, D. L., Cavalli-Sforza, L. L., Rabinowitz, D., McKusick, V. A. *Lancet*, 1968, ii, 194.
18. Daughaday, W. H., Kipnis, D. M. *Rec. Prog. Horm. Res.* 1966, **22**, 49.

CHAPTER FOUR

Reproductive Endocrinology

ALL aspects of reproduction depend on hormonal control. In the absence of pituitary gonadotrophins the gonads fail to develop completely, and removal of the pituitary in adult life causes reproductive failure. Control of gonadal development and generation of reproductive rhythms are among the major functions of the hypothalamic-pituitary system. Secretion of pituitary gonadotrophins causes gonadal differentiation and development, leading to maturation of germ-cells and secretion of gonadal steroid hormones. The gonadal steroids lead in turn to genital development and appropriate libido, being regulated in the female in a cyclic fashion which provides, repetitively and frequently, conditions suitable for conception and implantation. In addition, ovulation, implantation, and early development of the zygote are controlled by hormones, though fetal development becomes independent of pituitary and ovarian support when placental function is established.

Gonadal Function

The testis and ovary have two functional components—one secreting hormones, the other producing gametes. In the male, the interstitial or Leydig cells produce testosterone; in the female, the ovarian follicles secrete œstrogen, 17α OH-progesterone, and progesterone in varying amounts according to the time of the ovarian cycle. The small amounts of testosterone present in female blood are formed mainly by peripheral conversion from precursors, such as androstenedione, secreted by the ovary. The steroid hormones formed in the gonads and adrenals follow a common pattern of biosynthesis, with the exception of the 11β-hydroxylation characteristic of corticosteroid synthesis in the adrenal. These common pathways operate via the conversions summarised in fig. 10—from acetate to cholesterol, then to pregnenolone and its two major sets of derivatives, the Δ^5 and Δ^4 steroids arising from 17α OH-pregnenolone and 17α OH-progesterone respectively. Steroid hormones may either occur as intermediates in the synthetic pathways of a later product or as

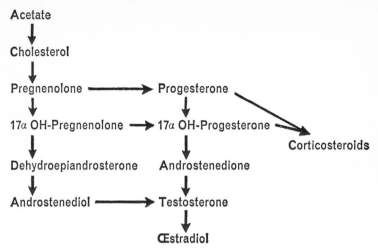

Fig. 10—Major steps in steroid biosynthesis.

end-products themselves: progesterone and testosterone, for example, may assume both of these roles.

The Testis

Spermatogenesis

The development of spermatozoa from the germinal epithelium proceeds by a series of cyclic changes in the spermatogonia, leading to the release of spermatozoa into the tubules after a maturation period of about 75 days. This development appears to depend on nutrition and hormonal activity by the surrounding Sertoli cells, which also phagocytise cytoplasmic residual bodies cast off by spermatids at the final stage of maturation. It has been suggested that these residual bodies supply the Sertoli cells with lipid, which is utilised in regulating the successive waves of sperm maturation.[1] About 10 million spermatozoa per gramme of testis are produced every day. While in the testis they are still immature in terms of metabolic activity, motility, and fertilising capacity. Further maturation occurs in the epididymis over a period of 10 days, and during contact with seminal plasma at ejaculation. The final modification (capacitation), which enables the spermatozoa to penetrate the zona pellucida of the ovum, takes place in the female genital tract. Of the 100 million or so sperms deposited during ejaculation, only a few hundred reach the ampulla of the tube, where fertilisation occurs.

In the testis F.S.H. promotes spermatogenesis and stimulates the metabolic activity of Sertoli cells. Both F.S.H. and testosterone are necessary for normal spermatogenesis. Although the Leydig cells are the main source of testosterone, there is evidence that this hormone is also synthesised in the germinal tubules,[2] probably by the Sertoli cells.[1] The feedback control of L.H. secretion in the male appears to operate via testosterone, but the regulation of F.S.H. secretion has not been clarified. Most studies show parallel variations in F.S.H. and L.H. in response to physiological stimuli. Although testosterone is not a potent inhibitor of F.S.H. secretion, œstradiol is extremely effective in suppressing F.S.H. release.[3] Tubular lesions and azoospermia are associated with high F.S.H. levels,[4] and a tubule hormone is thought to be involved in the negative feedback control of F.S.H. secretion under normal circumstances.

Leydig-cell Function[5]

Leydig cells comprise less than 10% of the testicular volume and secrete about 7 mg. of testosterone daily. Synthesis of testosterone from pregnenolone proceeds mainly via 17α OH-progesterone and androstenedione. At puberty, the rising secretion of pituitary L.H. favours the transformation of androstenedione to testosterone. The peripheral conversion of testosterone to œstrogen accounts for a large proportion of the œstradiol production in the male. Testosterone, the major androgen, originates almost entirely in the testis; the small amounts of ketosteroids secreted by the testis do not have significant androgenic activity, either directly or as precursors of testosterone. However, these and the much greater quantities of dehydroepiandrosterone (D.H.A.) secreted by the adrenal after puberty contribute substantially to urinary 17-ketosteroid excretion, which therefore cannot be used as a specific index of Leydig-cell activity. The best measure of androgen production is given by estimation of testosterone-secretion rate. For practical purposes, the measurement of plasma-testosterone levels by isotope derivative assay or binding assay provides a very useful indicator of androgen production in the male. Plasma-17α OH-progesterone level, measured by binding assay, and urinary œstrogen excretion measured by chemical assay may also provide useful indices of testis function.

In plasma, most of the circulating testosterone is bound to a specific carrier globulin, which transports both œstradiol and testosterone. This carrier protein is present in high concentrations in late pregnancy and during œstrogen treatment. It is not known whether the bound testosterone is biologically inactive, analogous to the bound fraction of plasma-cortisol, or whether it can affect responsive tissues. Testosterone is known to be converted in certain androgen-responsive tissues to a more potent androgen, dihydrotestosterone, which is localised in nuclei of target cells and appears to be the active intracellular androgen.[6] It has been proposed that testicular feminisation, a rare condition in which karyotypic males with testes and normal testosterone secretion show otherwise completely feminine external features, is due to defective conversion to dihydrotestosterone, resulting in failure of development of male secondary characteristics.[7]

The regulation of testis function depends entirely on the secretion of L.H. and F.S.H. by the pituitary gland. L.H. stimulates development and differentiation of the Leydig cells at puberty, leading to a 20-fold rise in plasma-testosterone. L.H. secretion is suppressed, rather slowly, by the feedback effects of testosterone and œstradiol on the hypothalamus. The predominant effect of L.H. on steroid synthesis in the testis is a rapid increase in testosterone secretion, mediated by cyclic A.M.P. and apparently due to accelerated conversion of cholesterol to pregnenolone in the mitochondria of the Leydig cells.

The Ovary[8]

The 7 million oocytes present in the ovary of the 30-week female fetus become enveloped by granulosa cells by about 40 weeks, forming follicles containing ova already in the prophase of meiotic division. These follicles undergo successive waves of development and atresia during fetal life and childhood, the number of primordial follicles falling from a maximum of 2 million just before birth to about 300,000 in the adult. The accumulation of atretic follicles forms much of the cortical stroma of the ovary, and neither ovulation nor corpus-luteum formation occurs before puberty. Cyclic secretion of gonadotrophins begins at puberty, leading to the full development of the adult ovary. The functional units, the follicles, each consist of an ovum and its two surrounding cell layers. The avascular inner layer of granulosa cells synthesises progesterone, which is secreted into the follicular fluid during the first half of the menstrual cycle, and which may also serve as precursor for œstrogen synthesis by the surrounding layer of theca-interna cells. Œstrogen is synthesised in the luteinised cells of the theca interna, predominantly via the Δ^5

pathway from pregenolone and 17 OH-progesterone, but also from progesterone produced by the granulosa cells. The theca interna is heavily luteinised and vascular during the first half of the cycle, and the synthesis and secretion of 17 OH-progesterone and œstradiol into the circulation reflect the predominant hormonal activity of the follicle—œstrogen secretion.

Although the earliest stages of follicle development seem to be independent of gonadotrophic activity, the mature follicle, with antral cavity surrounded by granulosa cells and the vascular theca layer, is responsive to gonadotrophic stimulation. F.S.H. initiates the development of a group of follicles, one of which matures and becomes responsive to the ovulatory stimulus of L.H. At ovulation, the ovum and surrounding cumulus of cells is extruded. Œstradiol secretion temporarily falls, then rises again during the luteal phase. The granulosa layer becomes vascularised and intensely luteinised, forming the yellow corpus luteum, which secretes up to 20 mg. of progesterone daily and involutes after about 2 weeks unless supported by the stimulus of chorionic gonadotrophin secreted by the trophoblast of an embedded zygote.

The ovum released at mid-cycle is viable for only about 12 hours; once fertilised, the zygote remains free for a further 5–6 days before implanting into the endometrium, which has been prepared by the actions of progesterone and œstradiol secreted by the corpus luteum. If implantation occurs, vascularisation of the developing zygote becomes established by the 9th day, and chorionic gonadotrophin is secreted into the maternal circulation, providing the stimulus for continued development of the corpus luteum. If implantation does not occur, the corpus luteum ceases to function after 12 days, and menstruation follows. The development and decline of the corpus luteum is paralleled by the rise and fall in the secretion of progesterone, 17α OH-progesterone, and œstradiol.

Fertilisation and Implantation

After ovulation, the ovum is captured by the fimbria of the fallopian tube and migrates quickly to the ampullary-isthmic junction. Here, fertilisation occurs a few hours later if spermatozoa have been recently deposited in the genital tract. The fertilised ovum then remains in the fallopian tube for about 4 days, and enters the uterus when developing from morula to early blastocyst. The timing of entry of the zygote into the uterus is very important; if it happens too early, implantation does not occur and ova are rapidly lost from the uterus. The transport of ova down the fallopian tube is influenced considerably by œstrogen—in a number of species it can be accelerated or delayed by varying doses of œstrogens. The commonest effect is accelerated transport, with premature arrival in the uterus and loss of the ovum.[9] The postovulatory decline in œstrogen levels may have a functional significance, in that maintained high levels would not be compatible with the normal period of tubal delay. The sharp decline in plasma-œstradiol levels which follows ovulation is clearly visible in fig. 11. When large doses of œstrogen are given for 3 days after intercourse, pregnancy does not occur, and the basis of this effect is most likely accelerated transport and loss of any zygote which may be present.

The human ovary contains millions of primary oocytes, of which only about 400 undergo the first maturation division to form the secondary oocyte at the time of ovulation. The second maturation division, which forms the mature ovum, does not occur until after penetration by sperm. Metabolic activity, protein synthesis, and R.N.A. synthesis in the ovum increase considerably after fertilisation, followed by enhanced D.N.A. synthesis before cell-division. The first division of the zygote occurs about 30 minutes after sperm penetration, and the second division 3 hours later. The morula stage, with up to 50 cells, becomes differentiated into the blastocyst at the time of entering the uterus. In later blastocysts, trophoblast cells begin to differentiate in preparation for implantation.

The endometrium must be suitably prepared by appropriate levels and timing of œstrogen and progesterone secreted by the corpus luteum. The trophoblast is extremely invasive and appears to be controlled by the decidual tissue of the endometrium. Once established, the trophoblast begins to secrete increasing quantities of chorionic gonadotrophin into the maternal circulation, stimulating the corpus luteum to increased secretion of œstrogen and progesterone, and maintaining its function during the first months of pregnancy. The presence of chorionic gonadotrophin in plasma and urine can be detected by radioimmunoassay as early as 8–10 days after ovulation[10]; the plasma-level rises steeply to reach a maximum 60 days after the last menstrual period, then drops after 2 weeks to lower levels for the remaining months of pregnancy. The precise role of chorionic gonadotrophin in pregnancy is not clear, for oophorectomy in early pregnancy does not commonly result in abortion. The corpus luteum is not, therefore, necessary for the continuation of pregnancy, and the functions of the large quantities of H.C.G. secreted during the second and third months of pregnancy remain obscure.

Measurement of Gonadotrophic and Gonadal Hormones

Enough gonadotrophin is excreted in urine to allow bioassay of F.S.H. and L.H., but the methods are demanding and barely sensitive enough to allow daily measurements. Radioimmunoassays for L.H. and F.S.H. are equally demanding but are sensitive enough to allow measurement of gonadotrophins in blood. These immunological procedures need to be carefully validated with regard to cross-reactions between L.H., F.S.H., T.S.H., and H.C.G., and suitably specific antisera must be used. Also, the pituitary and urinary forms of the hormones may differ in immunoreactivity, so that standards have to be chosen carefully. Antiserum to H.C.G. has been widely used for plasma-L.H. assays, sometimes with urinary L.H. reference standards. The current trend is towards the use of pituitary materials in systems for assays of pituitary extracts and serum samples, and urinary preparations for assays on gonadotrophins in urine.

Gonadal hormones have been measured in urine by chemical and isotopic methods of steroid assay, and in plasma by isotopic and protein-binding assays. Recently, the ability to produce antibodies to steroid-protein conjugates has been applied to radioimmunoassay of steroids in plasma. Assays for measurement of gonadotrophic and gonadal hormones in plasma are sensitive but not always very precise. This lack of precision has not been a major problem with L.H., but has led to conflicting notions about F.S.H. levels in plasma. Basal levels in normal subjects are not far above the noise level of some radioimmunoassay procedures.

Control of Ovulation[11]

All female mammals have an œstrous or menstrual cycle of reproductive activity. In some species (e.g., rabbit, cat, ferret) ovulation occurs as a central-nervous reflex after coitus, causing discharge of gonadotrophin from the pituitary. In the majority of mammals the central stimulus to ovulation is affected to only a minor degree by environmental stimuli, being primarily regulated by an internal hormone cycle mediated by a hypothalamic clock of characteristic frequency—e.g., 4 days in rats, 28 days in women. The potential for developing cyclical hypothalamic control systems for gonadotrophin release is present in both sexes during fetal life. In the male, androgen secretion from the fetal testis abolishes the intrinsic cyclicity of the hypothalamus, leading to the steady release of gonadotrophins from the pituitary during adult life. The menstrual bleeding of primates is an external marker of the end of the ovarian cycle and is due to endometrial necrosis and shedding following withdrawal of ovarian-hormone support for the vascular hypertrophic endometrium characteristic of the luteal phase of the cycle.

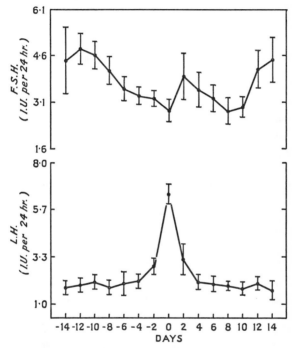

Fig. 11—Urinary excretion of F.S.H. and L.H. biological activity (mean ± S.E.M.) during 64 menstrual cycles.

The data are shown in relation to the L.H. peak at mid-cycle. (After Stevens.[13])

The integration of events in the menstrual cycle results from a series of interactions between hypothalamic, pituitary, and ovarian factors, producing the characteristic sequence of follicular development, ovulation, corpus-luteum formation, and menstruation or pregnancy.

The basic hormone patterns of the menstrual cycle were shown clearly by early studies on urinary excretion of gonadotrophin, pregnanediol, and œstrogen metabolites.[12] Œstrogen production rose during the preovulatory or follicular phase to reach a peak at the mid-cycle, falling then to lower levels and rising again during the postovulatory or luteal phase, and returning to low levels during the ensuing menstruation. On the other hand, pregnanediol, the major metabolite of progesterone, was low throughout the follicular phase, rising after mid-cycle to give a luteal-phase peak which has long been considered characteristic of an ovulatory cycle and adequate corpus-luteum function. Analysis of these early studies led to the conclusion that œstrogen excretion began to rise earlier than gonadotrophins and probably reached peak values before the mid-cycle peak of gonadotrophin excretion. The results of specific bioassays for L.H. and F.S.H. in urine have shown clearcut elevation of L.H. excretion at mid-cycle[13] (fig. 11). The pattern of F.S.H. excretion is extremely significant in relation to the control of follicular development. The early rise, followed by a decline until mid-cycle and the second nadir during the luteal phase, are consistent with studies on plasma-F.S.H. levels and provide support for current notions about the hormonal control of ovulation. More recent studies on plasma-gonadotrophin levels and urinary steroid-hormone excretion have confirmed the observation that œstradiol precedes and possibly stimulates L.H. release, clearly demonstrating that œstrogen excretion rises some days before the mid-cycle L.H. peak, with peak values on the day of the L.H. peak or 1–2 days beforehand.[14] Analysis of fractionated urinary œstrogen and progesterone metabolites in relation to plasma F.S.H. and L.H. levels have shown that a peak of urinary œstradiol invariably occurs on the day before the plasma-L.H. peak, whereas the peaks of the other major œstrogen metabolites (œstrone and œstriol) show a similar pattern with somewhat greater variability[15] (fig. 12). Such observations have been interpreted as meaning that the mid-cycle surge of gonadotrophin is caused by a preceding rise in œstradiol secretion. Support for this notion is provided by the demonstration that œstradiol injection stimulates L.H. release in anœstrous and oophorec-tomised ewes[16] (fig. 13). In these studies the minimum effective dose of infused œstradiol has been estimated to be comparable to that secreted by the sheep ovary during œstrus. More recently, œstrogen administration has been shown to cause L.H. release in rodents, monkeys, and women, usually after a preceding period of L.H. suppression. Under certain conditions, only the L.H.-suppressing effect of œstrogen is observed, but administration of adequate dosage and

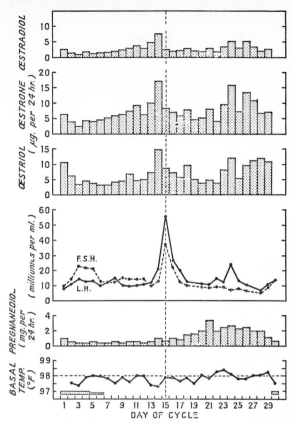

Fig. 12—*Œstrogen and pregnanediol excretion in urine during the menstrual cycle, compared with plasma-levels of F.S.H. and L.H. measured by radioimmunossay.* After Goebelsmann et al.[15]

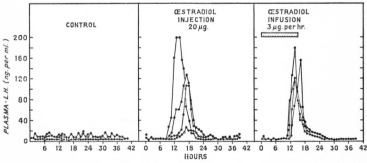

Fig. 13—*Stimulation of L.H. release in the sheep by intramuscular and intravenous administration of œstradiol 17β.* After Goding et al.[16]

duration has been shown to stimulate the secretion of L.H. as peaks similar to those which occur before ovulation.

The introduction of binding assays sensitive and specific enough to measure plasma-steroids has allowed more detailed analysis of the relationship between circulating steroid and gonadotrophin levels during the critical phases of the menstrual cycle. The accumulated knowledge about plasma-levels of L.H., F.S.H., œstradiol, progesterone, and 17α OH-progesterone can be summarised as follows:

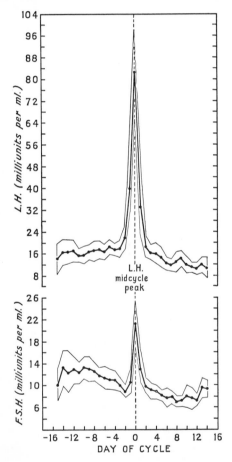

Fig. 14—Patterns of L.H. and F.S.H. secretion as shown by plasma-levels during 16 normal menstrual cycles.

Results are centred on the mid-cycle L.H. peak, and outer lines indicate 95% confidence limits of the means. (After Ross et al.[17])

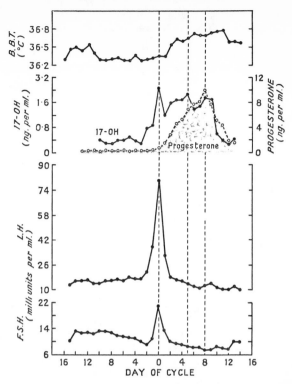

Fig. 15—Mean basal body temperature, plasma-17-hydroxyprogesterone and progesterone levels, and plasma L.H. and F.S.H. levels during 16 normal menstrual cycles.

After Ross et al.[17]

1. L.H. and F.S.H. both show prominent mid-cycle peaks, the L.H. peak being larger and more consistent. The significance of values observed at other times of the cycle has been more difficult to define, since they are not far above the minimum detectable limits of some assay procedures. However, the pooling and analysis of data derived from many cycles has shown[17] that mean plasma-L.H. levels begin to rise during the second part of the follicular phase, then rise sharply to reach about 5 times the basal level, fall rapidly within a day, often in a biphasic fashion, and decline again during the luteal phase. Pooled data have also shown that mean plasma-F.S.H. levels increase during the first few days of the follicular phase, then decline during the second part of the follicular phase to a preovulatory nadir just before the L.H. peak. Then follows an abrupt peak of plasma-F.S.H., coinciding with the L.H. peak, and a gradual decline to a luteal nadir about 10 days later, reaching the lowest levels of the cycle. After this luteal nadir, a slight rise occurs around the onset

of menses, possibly the beginning of the early follicular F.S.H. rise of the ensuing cycle (fig. 14). There is excellent agreement between this pattern and that obtained by bioassay of urinary F.S.H. and L.H. levels throughout the cycle (fig. 11).

2. Plasma-progesterone levels remain low throughout the follicular phase, rising at the time of the L.H. peak and reaching maximum levels about 8 days later, before declining again to levels close to those of the follicular phase (fig. 15). The postovulatory rise of progesterone was accompanied by progressive rise of basal body temperature, which became significant 4 days after the L.H. peak and remained elevated for about 9 days. The observed increase in progesterone secretion occurred while plasma L.H. and F.S.H. levels were falling, and the maximum level corresponded to the nadir of plasma F.S.H. Thus, the rising biosynthesis of progesterone does not depend on increased F.S.H. and L.H. secretion during the luteal phase and may in fact be partly responsible for the luteal decline in F.S.H. and L.H.

3. Plasma-17α OH-progesterone secretion has been shown to rise before and during the L.H. peak and has been thought to provide a measure of follicular maturation.[17] This steroid, the precursor of urinary pregnanetriol, begins to rise in plasma during the second part of the follicular phase, reaching a maximum coinciding with the L.H. peak. The plasma-level declines for several days after the L.H. peak, then rises again coincident with the profile of plasma-progesterone concentration and falls sharply just before the onset of menses. The highest levels of progesterone and 17α OH-progesterone occur at a time of declining levels of F.S.H. and L.H., the F.S.H. reaching its lowest levels at this time and thereafter beginning an early rise as progesterone levels decline again before the onset of the menses (fig. 15).

4. Plasma-œstradiol levels, measured by double isotope and binding assays, have been shown to be significantly related to the previously observed fluctuations in plasma-gonadotrophin levels.[18] From very low values during menstruation, plasma-œstradiol rises gradually during the early follicular phase, then sharply during the late follicular phase to reach very high levels immediately before the L.H. peak, falling again suddenly to much lower values at the time of ovulation. Œstradiol secretion then rises again to a luteal peak, followed by a further decline before the onset of menstruation (fig. 16). While some studies have shown that plasma œstradiol and L.H. levels reach a peak on the same day, most have shown that œstradiol reaches a peak before L.H. release occurs, so that the L.H. peak may occur at a time of falling œstradiol levels. Œstradiol reaches a high concentration immediately before the L.H. peak, and the role of œstrogen secretion in stimulating L.H. release seems well founded. Œstradiol secretion seems to precede 17α OH-progesterone secretion, then rises with it to a maximum at mid-cycle, being possibly responsible for the low level of F.S.H. which occurs immediately before the L.H. peak when œstradiol and 17α OH-progesterone levels are approaching their first maxima. The steady rise in plasma-L.H. before the main peak is probably due to stimulation by œstradiol secreted from

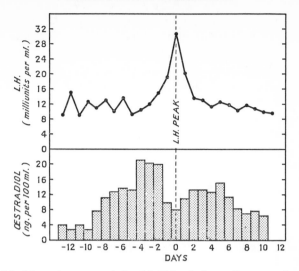

Fig. 16—Mean plasma œstradiol and L.H. levels during 12 menstrual cycles.
Œstradiol reaches a peak and begins to fall before L.H. peak occurs. (After Dufau et al.[18])

the developing follicle. This initial rise of plasma-L.H. may in turn further stimulate follicular secretion of œstradiol, leading to a situation in which positive feedback culminates in an abrupt surge of L.H. release once a critical level of œstradiol has been reached.

Thus, hormonal control of the normal menstrual cycle can be understood in terms of these observations on the levels of hormones in plasma and the known actions of gonadal hormones on gonadotrophin secretion. It is physiologically sound to refer such observations to the two important events of the cycle, the mid-cycle ovulatory release of L.H. and the ensuing menstrual flow which delineates the end of the cycle. The beginning of the cycle is much less simple to define but probably occurs during the antecedent cycle, just before menstruation. It is likely that the rise of F.S.H. which occurs after the decline of gonadal steroid levels at the end of the preceding luteal phase may initiate the next cycle of follicular maturation. This rise in F.S.H. secretion, together with the more constant release of L.H. by the pituitary, continues during the first part of the succeeding follicular phase, leading to rising œstradiol secretion which both suppresses F.S.H. secretion (thereby preventing development of other follicles) and stimulates L.H. secretion progressively over the last few days to lead, via positive feedback, to an explosive release of L.H. which stimulates ovulation and initiates luteinisation. The secretion of follicular steroids (œstradiol and 17α OH-progesterone) declines briefly following follicular rupture, possibly due to structural and vascular changes in the follicle, then rises and falls again in parallel with the secretion of progesterone by the corpus luteum. The high levels of corpus-luteum steroids suppress secretion of both F.S.H. and L.H. during the luteal phase, the decline in steroid secretion at luteal involution being followed by a rise in F.S.H. secretion which initiates the next cycle of follicular development.

Induction of Ovulation

Ovulation can be induced in infertile women by treatment with human gonadotrophin of pituitary or urinary origin, or by stimulation of endogenous gonadotrophin secretion with clomiphene. Treatment with human pituitary gonadotrophin was introduced by Gemzell, who showed that ovulation can be achieved in over 90% of suitable patients, and pregnancy in about 50%, by treatment with pituitary extracts rich in F.S.H.[19] Patients likely to respond to this treatment are those who have normal but non-functioning ovaries and low gonadotrophin secretion, as well as other features indicating potential fertility. Although failure of ovulation is the cause of only about 15% of cases of infertility, the group is important in being potentially curable by gonadotrophin or clomiphene therapy. When such patients are treated with human pituitary gonadotrophin (H.P.G.) under carefully controlled conditions, a high incidence of ovulation and pregnancy can be achieved. Good results have also been obtained by treatment with human menopausal gonadotrophin (H.M.G.) extracted from urine by the method of Donini to provide the preparation known as 'Pergonal'.

After initial treatment with an F.S.H.-rich gonadotrophin extract from pituitary or urine to stimulate follicle maturation, ovulation is triggered by a large dose of H.C.G., which has mainly L.H.-like actions. All preparations of gonadotrophin used for ovulation induction contain moderate quantities of L.H. in addition to the F.S.H. necessary for follicle stimulation. Since combined secretion of F.S.H. and L.H. appears necessary for normal follicle development and œstrogen secretion, the presence of L.H. in therapeutic preparations contributes to the ensuing ovarian response of follicular maturation. Quite wide variations in F.S.H./L.H. ratio seem to have relatively little influence on the effectiveness of the gonadotrophin preparations used for ovulation induction.

The complications of gonadotrophin administration include multiple pregnancy, and ovarian hyperstimulation with cyst formation and occasional systemic disturbances. Gemzell's results with gonadotrophin therapy have stimulated interest in defining optimum conditions of treatment. A major contribution to this aim has been provided by the development of a rapid assay method for urinary œstrogen, allowing daily estimations of œstrogen excretion to be made during treatment. Brown et al.[20] found that fertility is best achieved by graded treatment with gonadotrophin until œstrogen excretion is rising to within the range 50–100 μg. daily. At this time, a dose of 3000 units H.C.G. is given to induce ovulation, sometimes followed by further small doses during the luteal phase. Despite considerable differences in sensitivity between subjects, individual women show a fairly reproducible pattern of response to H.C.G., which enables the optimum dosage to be attained by repeated courses of treatment. It seems likely that the incidence of multiple pregnancy is related to excessive ovulating doses of H.C.G. and that careful control of treatment should reduce the incidence of overstimulation. In a group of 45 women treated for 229 cycles by Brown and his colleagues,[20] ovulation was achieved in all, and the pregnancy rate was 90%. An initial incidence of 26% for multiple births was expected to be reduced by careful adjustment of H.C.G. dosage.

Gonadotrophin therapy requires careful monitoring of both dosage and response to treatment, for patients' requirements have been known to cover a 32-fold range.[21] In some cases a single injection of F.S.H., followed several days later by H.C.G., has resulted in pregnancy, demonstrating clearly the ability of the follicle to undergo maturation after an initial stimulus. Studies on the addition of H.C.G. (which has an L.H.-like action) to F.S.H. treatment have shown a significant increase in œstrogen excretion, consistent with the proposal that L.H. may act synergistically with F.S.H. to promote œstrogen secretion by the developing follicle.

Urinary gonadotrophin assay is useful in the selection of patients. Women with ovarian failure have high urinary gonadotrophin levels characteristic of the postmenopausal state. Very low levels are found in some women with pituitary or hypothalamic lesions, but most infertile patients have normal basal urinary levels without the cyclic variations of normal hypothalamic control. In general, exogenous gonadotrophin therapy is most suitable for patients with deficient gonadotrophin secretion and should be reserved for patients who are unresponsive to stimulation of endogenous gonadotrophin release.

L.H. release can be stimulated by œstrogen treatment, but because of lack of responsiveness of the ovary this rarely leads to ovulation and pregnancy. However, administration of an anti-œstrogen, clomiphene citrate, has often been followed by induction of ovulation and pregnancy. Treatment with clomiphene for a few days produces a striking increase in œstrogen secretion by the ovary and a rise in L.H. and F.S.H. secretion. After cessation of treatment, L.H. levels drop then rise again to high values a few days later.

The action of clomiphene depends mainly on competition with œstrogen at the hypothalamic level, causing increased F.S.H. and L.H. release. These hormones act on the follicles, possibly aided by a local action of clomiphene in the ovary, causing follicular development with increasing œstrogen secretion which finally takes off into positive feedback to the hypothalamus, to trigger a spurt of L.H. release. In this situation a suitably primed follicle is present in the ovary and ovulation frequently occurs. In a series of 2616 patients treated with clomiphene, ovulation occurred in 70%, of whom 40% became pregnant.[22] Multiple pregnancies occur in about 6% of cases, and severe ovarian hyperstimulation is rare. Patients with the polycystic ovary syndrome (Stein-Leventhal syndrome) are very sensitive to clomiphene therapy, ovulation being achieved in 95% and pregnancy in up to 50%. The most common side-effects of clomiphene are ovarian enlargement and hot flushes, the latter being a manifestation of the compound's anti-œstrogenic effect.

Hormonal Contraception

Oral œstrogen-progestagen combinations provide the most effective method of fertility control apart from sterilisation. Since their introduction in 1956, these steroidal contraceptives have been taken by millions of women over periods of several years, and precise figures on their efficacy and hazards are now becoming available. The failure-rate of oral contraceptives is very low, as shown by the pregnancy incidence of only 1 per 1000 woman-years of use (in contrast to more than 800 pregnancies without contraception). Combined oral contraceptives act primarily by suppressing ovulation. The mid-cycle L.H. peak is abolished by progestational compounds through feedback inhibition. F.S.H. secretion is inhibited by the œstrogenic component of oral contraceptives, leading in turn to failure of follicular development and œstradiol secretion. Thus, the action of the combined preparations is due to two effects: (i) inhibition of follicle ripening by suppression of F.S.H. secretion, and (ii) abolition of the L.H. peak by inhibition of the release mechanism at the hypothalamic level, as well as suppression of the usual feedback stimulus to L.H. release by œstradiol secreted from the developing follicle.[18] This hormonal checkmate leaves the ovary in a quiescent state, and causes reduction in both activity and size of the ovary.

Other effects of steroidal contraceptives on cervical mucus and sperm activity have been described, but clearly they act mainly on ovulation. Suppression of ovulation over a period of several years is not associated with an extension of potential reproductive life, for the natural rate of follicle atresia continues steadily, and ovarian failure occurs as usual in middle age. The continued use of combined oral contraceptives is associated with small but definite risks to life, mainly from venous thromboembolism and cerebral thrombosis. Less severe reactions are seen in the occasional development of jaundice and the rare occurrence of severe hypertension. Disorders of carbohydrate and lipid metabolism can also be demonstrated in a significant proportion of women using oral contraceptives. Despite this imposing list of complications, it is important to recognise that the risks of oral contraception are considerably lower than any of those associated with abortion, pregnancy, road accidents, smoking, and drinking.[23] Most dangers of prolonged oral contraception are due to the œstrogenic component, and more attention is now being given to the use of progestagens alone for contraception.

Progestagens, such as chlormadinone, have given less effective fertility control than combined preparations containing œstrogen. Progestagens cause changes in the cervical mucus and inhibit sperm penetration, but they do not suppress ovulation. Long-term progestagen treatment with depot injections, silastic implants, or pessaries impregnated with progestagen have also been examined as possible alternatives to the combined preparations. The appearance of mammary nodules in dogs being tested for long-term effects of chlormadinone has caused anxiety about its neoplastic potential in women, though the possibility appears remote.

Further developments in the hormonal control of fertility will be increasingly concerned with agents which interfere with implantation or development of the fertilised ovum. Work with antibodies to œstradiol has confirmed that œstradiol secretion is essential for implantation of the ovum in the rat.[23] In women the luteal rise in œstrogen and progesterone secretion is probably necessary for implantation, and the use of anti-œstrogens and anti-progestagens may offer useful alternatives to pituitary-hormone blockade. The control of male fertility has received little attention, despite the equal susceptibility of the male gonads to inhibition by hormonal methods. The use of œstrogen-androgen combinations has been proposed for suppression of F.S.H. release and inhibition of spermatogenesis with retention of normal libido[1] but is unlikely to gain popular acceptance because it reduces testicular size, analogous to the effect of œtrogen-prcgestagen contraceptives in the ovary.

Various chemicals have a direct suppressant action on spermatozoa, without influencing endocrine function.[24] Unfortunately, the most promising of these also has an 'Antabuse'-like effect when alcohol is taken. The traditional attitude that ingestion of contraceptives should be the female's responsibility alone is unlikely to persist, but any antispermatogenic chemicals developed must be proved to cause sterilisation without risk of genetic damage. Some simple compounds, such as a chlorinated derivative of glycerol, have been reported to produce striking inhibition of epididymal sperm development.

1. Lacy, D., Pettit, J. A. *Br. med. Bull.* 1970, **26**, 87.
2. Dufau, M. L., DeKretzer, D. M., Hudson, B. *Endocrinology*, 1971, **88**, 825.
3. McCullagh, E. P., Hruby, F. J. *J. clin. Endocr. Metab.* 1949, **9**, 113.
4. Franchimont, P. *in* Advances in the Biosciences (edited by G. Raspe); p. 19. Vieweg, 1967.
5. Lipsett, M. B. *in* Diseases of Metabolism (edited by P. K. Bondy); p. 1171. Philadelphia, 1969.
6. Bruchovsky, N., Wilson, J. D. *J. biol. Chem.* 1968, **243**, 2012.
7. Northcutt, R. C., Island, D. P., Liddle, G. W. *J. clin. Endocr.* 1969, **29**, 422.
8. Kase, N. G. *in* Diseases of Metabolism (edited by P. K. Bondy); p. 1191. Philadelphia, 1969.
9. Greenwald, G. S. *in* Progress in Infertility (edited by S. J. Behrman and R. W. Kistner); p. 157. Boston, 1968.
10. Wide, L. *Lancet*, 1969, ii, 863.
11. Harris, G. W., Naftolin, F. *Br. med. Bull.* 1970, **26**, 3.
12. Brown, J. B., Klopper, A., Loraine, J. A. *J. Endocr.* 1958, **17**, 401.
13. Stevens, V. C. *in* Recent Research on Gonadotrophic Hormones (edited by E. T. Bell and J. A. Loraine); p. 227. Edinburgh, 1967.

4. Burger, H. G., Catt, K. J., Brown, J. B. *J. clin. Endocr.* 1968, **28**, 1508.
15. Goebelsmann, U., Midgley, A. R., Jaffe, R. B. *ibid.* 1969, **29**, 1222.
16. Goding, J. R., Catt, K. J., Brown, J. M., Kaltenbach, C. C., Cumming, I. A., Mole, B. J. *Endocrinology*, 1969, **85**, 133.
17. Ross, G. T., Cargille, C. M., Lipsett, M. B., Rayford, P. L., Marshall, J. R., Strott, C. A., Rodbard, D. Gregory Pincus Memorial Lecture. Laurentian Hormone Conference 1969 (in the press).
8. Dufau, M., Catt, K. J., Dulmanis, A., Fullerton, M., Hudson, B., Burger, H. G. *Lancet*, 1970, i, 271.
19. Gemzell, C. A., Roos, P., Loeffler, F. E. *in* Progress in Infertility (edited by S. J. Behrman and R. W. Kistner); p. 375. Boston, 1968.
20. Brown, J. B., Evans, J. H., Adey, F. D., Taft, H. P., Townsend, L. *J. Obstet. Gynæc. Br. Commonw.* 1969, **76**, 289.
21. Crooke, A. C. *Br. med. Bull.* 1970, **26**, 17.
22. Kistner, R. W. *in* Progress in Infertility (edited by S. J. Behrman and R. W. Kistner); p. 407. Boston, 1968.
23. Ferin, M., Zimmering, P. E., VandeWiele, R. L. *Endocrinology*, 1969, **84**, 893.
24. Jackson, H. *Br. med. Bull.* 1970, **26**, 85.

CHAPTER FIVE

Adrenal Cortex

WHEREAS endocrine glands derived in embryological development from the gut and related structures characteristically secrete peptide hormones which act upon cell-membrane receptors, glands arising from mesodermal origins secrete steroid hormones which act upon receptors in the nuclei of responsive cells. Peptide hormones are complex structures and have relatively few features in common except for their basic composition of aminoacids. They are water soluble and circulate in blood without association with other proteins. All steroid hormones are of basically similar structure, with relatively minor chemical differences which lead to striking alterations in biological activity. They are sparingly soluble in water, and usually circulate in association with binding proteins in plasma. The characteristic structure of steroid hormones is that of a relatively flat four-membered ring group carrying attached functional groups (-H, -CH$_3$, -OH, $=$ O) which project above (β) or below (α) the plane of the ring structure. Although numerous variations of structure occur in the precursors and metabolites of the active steroid hormones, the configurations of the major steroids are relatively few and quite well defined (fig. 17). Despite these apparently minor differences among the steroids, their individual molecular configurations confer moderate specificity in their ability to react with transport proteins, and high specificity in their reaction with nuclear receptors in target cells. The biosynthetic pathways for steroid formation are closely similar in the various steroid-producing tissues, which are characterised by the predominant secretion of one particular steroid molecule according to the spectrum of enyzme activity present in the tissue, and smaller quantities of steroids more characteristic of other tissues. Thus, the adrenal secretes small quantities of testosterone and œstradiol, small amounts of œstradiol are produced in the testis, and traces of testosterone are produced in the ovary. The characteristic enzymes for corticosteroid synthesis are not present in the gonads, and all glucocorticoid and mineralocorticoid production takes place in the adrenal cortex.

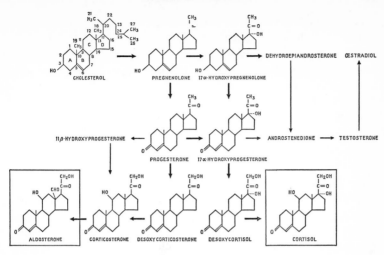

Fig. 17—Biosynthetic pathways in the adrenal gland to the major steroid hormones—cortisol and aldosterone.
Structures of the more important intermediates are shown.

The secretion of steroid hormones by the adrenal cortex involves biosynthetic pathways leading from cholesterol through progesterone and 17α OH-progesterone to the two major adrenal steroids, cortisol (hydrocortisone or compound F) and aldosterone (fig. 17). Cortisol is the major glucocorticoid of primates and certain other species (sheep, cow, cat, dog) whereas corticosterone is the predominant glucocorticoid secreted by the adrenal in rodents. The major minera-

TABLE II—STEROID SECRETION BY HUMAN ADRENAL

Steroid	Daily secretion-rate
Cortisol	8–25 mg. (14 mg.)
Corticosterone	2–4 mg.
Aldosterone	50–200 μg. (100 μg.)
Dehydroepiandrosterone	15–30 mg. (20 mg.)
Progesterone	0·4–0·8 mg.
Androstenedione	1–10 mg.
Testosterone	Trace
Œstradiol	Trace

About 50 steroids have been isolated from the adrenal cortex. Most are inactive precursors of the major steroids secreted into the adrenal vein.

locorticoid is aldosterone in almost all species, though certain glucocorticoids exhibit a degree of mineralocorticoid activity. In man,
several other steroids are secreted by the adrenal (table II), including
small amounts of progesterone, testosterone, and œstrogen, and
larger quantities of 17-ketosteroids, mainly as dehydroepiandrosterone (D.H.A.). The sex hormones secreted by the adrenal are not
normally of biological significance compared with those arising from
the gonads, though adrenal androgen secretion has been implicated
in pubertal hair growth and maintenace of libido in the female.

Biological Effects of Steroid Hormones

These may be considered at several levels of cellular organisation,
ranging from the pathological results of deficiency or excess in the
whole animal, through physiological effects and biochemical actions,
to biophysical interactions with nuclear components. The well-
known effects of adrenal-steroid deficiency include sodium loss,
potassium retention, decrease in blood-volume, liver glycogen, and
blood-sugar, and impairment of renal function with reduced excretion of water, ammonia, and urea. This combination of features
results from simultaneous disturbances of intermediary metabolism,
especially gluconeogenesis, and of mineral metabolism, especially
sodium handling. The opposite situation of steroid excess is seen
most frequently as a picture of predominant glucocorticoid excess,
due to Cushing's syndrome or steroid therapy. Here, protein catabolism is prominent, manifested by atrophy of skin, muscle, and
bone matrix; enhanced gluconeogenesis and glycogen deposition are
characteristic, and striking atrophy of lymphoid tissue occurs. Some
degree of mineralocorticoid activity occurs in these conditions,
causing sodium retention and its consequences. However, the picture
of mineralocorticoid excess is seen in pure form in patients with
aldosterone-secreting tumours, resulting in hypokalæmic alkalosis and
sodium retention, with relatively minor disturbances of carbohydrate
metabolism.

The major effects of glucocorticoids upon intermediary metabolism
are to increase the conversion of endogenous protein to carbohydrate
and to promote glycogen storage in the liver.[1] Adrenalectomised
animals cannot meet demands for glucose by conversion of protein
to carbohydrate, and depend upon regular feeding for glucose
homœostasis. The biochemical basis of this action of glucocorticoids is the stimulation of synthesis of liver enzymes concerned with

transformation of protein into carbohydrates. The activities of enzymes concerned with aminoacid degradation, urea metabolism, and transamination are increased by corticosteroid treatment. This stimulation of enzyme activity is due to increased enzyme synthesis, brought about by enhanced transcription of D.N.A. to provide further messenger R.N.A. for synthesis of specific enzymes. This action of glucocorticoids involves reaction of the molecule with specific nuclear components, causing unlocking or exposure of critical D.N.A. sequences responsible for formation of specific messenger R.N.A. molecules.

The effects of mineralocorticoids on sodium handling are also due to an ultimate action on nuclear chromatin, causing increased messenger R.N.A. (mR.N.A.) formation and new protein synthesis in responsive cells of the kidney and bladder epithelium.[2] The action of the specific protein synthesis induced by aldosterone is not yet clear, but it results in elevated sodium transport by the stimulated cell. In the kidney, aldosterone stimulates sodium reabsorption in the distal tubule, and simultaneous secretion of potassium and hydrogen ions. The effects of aldosterone on sodium and potassium handling are not confined to the renal tubule; similar actions occur in salivary gland, sweat glands, and intestine, and an effect upon the proximal renal tubule has been described. During excessive aldosterone secretion, after a certain degree of sodium retention the kidney eventually "escapes" from the effect of aldosterone and no further sodium is retained. This happens by a readjustment of proximal tubular function leading to restoration of sodium balance at a higher extracellular-fluid volume than normal. Other aldosterone-responsive glands do not show this escape, and maintain an abnormally low sodium/potassium ratio in their secretions. The distal tubule also does not escape from the action of aldosterone, since the increased excretion of potassium continues and a substantial negative potassium balance develops.

Adrenal Steroid Biosynthesis[3]

The histological zonation of the adrenal cortex is accompanied by a functional zonation of the enzymes concerned in hormone biosynthesis. Although the zonation is less clearcut in man than in some other species, there is good evidence that aldosterone secretion is largely confined to the zona glomerulosa and cortisol secretion to the zona fasciculata; in some species androgen synthesis occurs predominantly in the reticularis. Several of the biosynthetic steps in adrenal-steroid formation take place in the mitochondria, which have a vesicotubular structure and a large surface area compared with the laminar cristæ of mitochondria in other tissues. A.C.T.H. stimulation has predominant effects upon lipid content and mitochondrial morphology in the fasciculata, while mitochondria of the glomerulosa layer are more affected by sodium deficiency. The maintenance of adrenal mass is also thought to require G.H. secretion by the pituitary, but A.C.T.H. is the predominant factor. Mitotic activity is most striking in the glomerulosa, and the entire cortex can regenerate from the adrenal capsule remaining after removal of the inner zones of the gland.

Storage of steroid hormones within the adrenal is minimal, most of the lipid being present as cholesterol and cholesterol ester. These, together with plasma-cholesterol, provide the substrate for adrenal-steroid synthesis. The main steps in this biosynthetic pathway are well defined (fig. 17), commencing with the cleavage of the cholesterol side-chain by mitochondrial enzymes to form Δ^5-pregnenolone, the major precursor of all steroid hormones. There follows a conversion of pregnenolone to the Δ^4 3-ketosteriod configuration characteristic of progesterone and its derivatives, and a series of hydroxylation steps—at positions 17 and 21 in the microsomes, and position 11 in the mitochondria. The human adrenal is extremely active in 17-hydroxylation, and forms cortisol as the major glucocorticoid. In the zona glomerulosa, corticosterone undergoes 18-hydroxylation during biosynthetic conversion to aldosterone.

Two well-known features of adrenal steroid biosynthesis are the requirement for reduced N.A.D.P. for the various hydroxylations, and the decrease in ascorbic-acid levels in the adrenal after stimulation of steroidogenesis by A.C.T.H. The importance of an adequate supply of reduced N.A.P.D. for steroidogenesis has led to proposals that it may represent a site of action of A.C.T.H. on steroid synthesis. The ascorbic-acid depletion induced by A.C.T.H. was used by Sayers to establish a valuable bioassay for this peptide, but its exact relation to steroidogenesis has not been defined.

Regulation of Glucocorticoid Secretion

A.C.T.H. is responsible for the maintenance of adrenal structure and function, causing predominant stimulation of glucocorticoid secretion and exerting a permissive or supportive action on aldosterone secretion (i.e., necessary for aldosterone secretion but not the main stimulus). The 39-aminoacid A.C.T.H. peptide chain is secreted by specific basophil cells in response to C.R.F. formed in the hypothalamus and transported by the portal vessels to the anterior pituitary. Although C.R.F. was the first hypothalamic releasing factor to be defined, its structure has not yet been elucidated, though there is evidence that it is a small peptide.

C.R.F. acts rapidly on the pituitary, causing A.C.T.H. release within

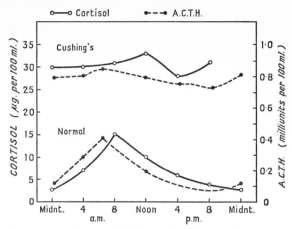

Fig. 18—Plasma cortisol and A.C.T.H. in a healthy individual and in a patient with Cushing's syndrome (from Glenn et al.[4]).

a minute or two. The normal secretion of A.C.T.H. is cyclical, leading to a circadian rhythm in steroid secretion by the adrenal, with very low plasma-cortisol levels near midnight and peak levels in the early morning (fig. 18). This 24-hour rhythmic secretion of A.C.T.H. and cortisol seems to be related to the sleep pattern, and can be modified by alterations in daily activity. The control mechanisms for A.C.T.H. secretion[5] operate through the hypothalamic centres responsible for C.R.F. formation (fig. 19). A simple reciprocal feedback system between plasma-cortisol and A.C.T.H. release seems to prevail under basal conditions, and is influenced by a related mechanism which determines the normal diurnal variation in A.C.T.H. secretion. A further independent system operates under various stressful situations to override the basal homœostatic control system, causing transient elevations of plasma-cortisol during acute stress such as trauma or infection. This responsiveness to acute stimuli forms the basis for various tests of pituitary-adrenal function, such as stimulation by A.C.T.H., pyrogen, hypoglycæmia, and metyrapone, which test the reserve capacity of the system. Also, the feedback mechanism provides the basis for suppression tests making use of potent synthetic glucocorticoids to inhibit A.C.T.H. release and adrenal steroid production, to distinguish between the various forms of corticosteroid hypersecretion by hyperplastic and neoplastic adrenal lesions.

The aminoacid sequence of A.C.T.H. has been determined in cow, pig, sheep, and man, and the porcine and human hormones have been

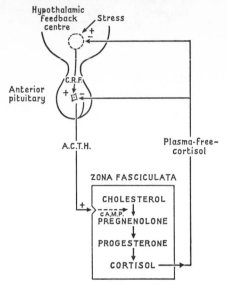

Fig. 19—Regulation of corticosteroid secretion.

In the hypothalamus, secretion of c.r.f. is influenced by negative feedback from the circulating free cortisol level, a mechanism imposing diurnal variation, and stressful stimuli mediated by the central nervous system. There is probably also direct feedback by cortisol to the corticotrophin-secreting cells in the anterior pituitary. a.c.t.h. secreted in response to these stimuli combines with membrane receptors on the zona fasciculata cells, leading to formation of cyclic a.m.p. which stimulates pregnenolone synthesis in the mitochondria.

completely synthesised. The sequences 1–24 and 34–39 are identical in all species studied, individual species differences appearing in the 25–33 region of the peptide chain. Biological activity is confined to the N-terminal portion of the molecule, the peptide 1–24 possessing the full activity of the native 1–39 molecule (fig. 20). The synthetic 1–24 peptide 'Synacthen' is of value for adrenal stimulation tests,

1	2	3	4		22	23	24	25	26		32	33	34	35	36	37	38	39
Ser-	Tyr-	Ser-	Met	---	Val-	Tyr-	Pro-	Asp-	Ala	---	Ala-	Glu-	Ala-	Phe-	Pro-	Leu-	Glu-	Phe

1-24	25-33	34-39
← Common to all species → Full biological activity M.S.H. activity Synthetic product	← Region of → species difference and immunological specificity	← Common to all species →

Fig. 20—A.C.T.H. molecule showing the regions of biological activity and species specificity.

and a modified version of the synthetic peptide containing unusual aminoacids has a prolonged action in man.[6] The intrinsic M.S.H. activity of corticotrophin is also present in the synthetic peptide, since similar residues occur within the first 13 residues of A.C.T.H. and those of the M.S.H. molecules. Although M.S.H. has only very minor functions in man, the pigmentation which accompanies hypersecretion of A.C.T.H. seems to be due to an associated oversecretion of M.S.H., rather than to the weak inherent M.S.H. activity of corticotrophin.

Action of A.C.T.H. on Adrenal

A.C.T.H. is responsible for maintenance of the structure, size, and vascularity of the adrenal cortex, and for the regulation of corticosteroid secretion.[7] The small quantity of A.C.T.H. secreted each day by the human pituitary maintains the average adrenal mass at about 13 g. and controls the synthesis of enzyme proteins responsible for the several steps of steroidogenesis. A.C.T.H. also acutely controls steroid-hormone secretion, and causes the normal cyclical secretion of cortisol throughout the day. The pituitary secretes A.C.T.H. intermittently as a series of pulses throughout the day, resulting in episodic secretion of cortisol with approximately half the daily production during the early-morning hours of sleep. Administration of A.C.T.H. causes lipid depletion and hyperplasia of mitochondria especially in the zona fasciculata, followed by hypertrophy of this layer. The manner in which A.C.T.H. exerts acute effects upon steroidogenesis has lately been partially elucidated. The hormone does not seem to enter the adrenal cells, but acts upon a membrane receptor site which is connected functionally with an adjacent adenyl-cyclase system leading to increased formation of cyclic A.M.P. This nucleotide acts upon R.N.A. to modulate the synthesis of a specific protein regulator molecule which is probably formed in the mitochondria. This labile protein promotes the utilisation of cholesterol for steroidogenesis, either by enhancing the transport of cholesterol from liposome to mitochondria, or by stimulating the side-chain cleavage reaction on the mitochondria. Whereas plasma-cholesterol is utilised by the adrenal for steroid biosynthesis under basal conditions, further stimulation by A.C.T.H. causes breakdown of stored cholesterol ester followed by increased utilisation of free cholesterol for corticosteroid synthesis. The steroids produced in response to A.C.T.H. are predominantly cortisol, corticosterone, and ketosteroids, with smaller amounts of androgen and œstrogen; aldosterone secretion shows an initial rise after A.C.T.H. then falls to low levels despite continued administration, while glucocorticoid secretion progressively increases.[8]

Regulation of Mineralocorticoid Secretion

Aldosterone secretion is closely correlated with salt metabolism, being elevated during sodium restriction and reduced by sodium loading, while the opposite changes are seen during alterations of potassium balance. The major role of aldosterone is to maintain sodium homœostasis, and the largest increases in aldosterone secretion occur under conditions of sodium depletion.

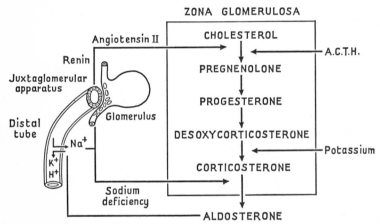

Fig. 21—Factors stimulating aldosterone secretion in the zona glomerulosa, showing loci at which the various factors act upon the aldosterone biosynthetic pathway.

The glomerulosa zone of the adrenal has long been known to be affected by altered sodium balance, and to show less atrophy than the fasciculata layer after hypophysectomy. The secretion of aldosterone by the glomerulosa cells in response to sodium deficiency and potassium excess has been demonstrated in numerous species, and the biosynthetic mechanism shown to proceed via 18-hydroxylation of corticosterone by mitochondrial enzyme systems.

The mechanism by which sodium depletion activates the zona glomerulosa is not yet clear, though several factors which can stimulate aldosterone secretion have been identified[9] (fig. 21);

A.C.T.H., angiotensin II, and elevated serum-potassium are potent stimuli, while reduction of plasma-sodium is less effective.

A.C.T.H. is not the major regulator of aldosterone secretion, but plays a supportive role in basal secretion and in the responsiveness to sodium depletion. Hypophysectomy and hypopituitarism are followed by a fall in aldosterone secretion and reduced response to salt deprivation. A.C.T.H. replacement corrects these defects, but administration of A.C.T.H. to healthy individuals causes a brief initial rise in aldosterone secretion followed by a fall. There is extensive experimental evidence that A.C.T.H. is not responsible for the acute changes of aldosterone secretion which accompany variations in sodium balance and blood-volume. Further, patients with adrenal hyperplasia due to excess A.C.T.H. secretion almost never show elevated aldosterone secretion.

Renin-angiotensin System

Renin is an enzyme produced in the cells of the juxtaglomerular apparatus, a complex structure formed by the apposition of the macula densa region of the distal convoluted tubule and the cells of the afferent arteriole supplying the corresponding glomerulus. This arrangement seems primarily concerned with sodium handling, via local regulation of glomerular blood-flow and tubule function in response to changes in electrolyte composition and concentration of tubular fluid. Little is known about the nature of this intrarenal regulation, but the secretion of renin into the general circulation and its actions have been exhaustively studied and clarified[10] (fig. 22). Release of renin is stimulated by sodium depletion and decreased intravascular volume, and is inhibited by volume expansion. The enzyme acts upon a plasma globulin (renin substrate) to cleave off a decapeptide (angiotensin I) which is converted to an octapeptide (angiotensin II) during passage through the lung and kidney. Angiotensin II is an extremely powerful vasoconstrictor, and stimulates aldosterone secretion by the adrenal cortex in man and several other species. Although angiotensin II is probably not concerned in normal blood-pressure regulation, excessive angiotension production may contribute to the hypertension of human renal disease. The physiological role of the renin-angiotensin-aldosterone system in normal aldosterone regulation is controversial, since certain experimental data conflict with the earlier notion that it is the main controlling factor—e.g., not all species show a sustained aldosterone response to angiotensin II (sheep), or even a good response (rat); dissociation of angiotensin II and aldosterone levels occurs under certain circumstances (correction of sodium deficiency, oral-contraceptive therapy); and angiotensin II does not mimic the biosynthetic effect of sodium-ion deficiency upon aldosterone formation from corticosterone.[1] However, there are several human disorders accompanied by increased renin-angiotensin activity and high

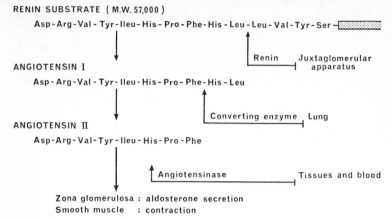

RENIN SUBSTRATE (M.W. 57,000)

Asp-Arg-Val-Tyr-Ileu-His-Pro-Phe-His-Leu-Leu-Val-Tyr-Ser

ANGIOTENSIN I

Asp-Arg-Val-Tyr-Ileu-His-Pro-Phe-His-Leu

Renin   Juxtaglomerular apparatus

ANGIOTENSIN II

Asp-Arg-Val-Tyr-Ileu-His-Pro-Phe

Converting enzyme   Lung

Angiotensinase   Tissues and blood

Zona glomerulosa : aldosterone secretion
Smooth muscle   : contraction

Fig. 22—Renin-angiotensin system.

Angiotensin II has a half-life in the circulation of only one minute, being rapidly metabolised to inactive peptides by angiotensinase in peripheral vascular beds. Although angiotensin II can exert potent actions on vascular smooth muscle and aldosterone secretion, the extent to which these actions operate under physiological conditions is uncertain.

The majority of cortisol and corticosterone is normally bound to transcortin (C.B.G.) and albumin.

aldosterone secretion (e.g., cirrhosis with ascites, nephrotic syndrome, malignant hypertension, and renovascular disease) in which a stimulating effect of angiotensin II on aldosterone secretion seems likely. In primary aldosteronism, characterised by excess aldosterone secretion from an adrenal adenoma, the resulting sodium retention and volume expansion leads to suppression of renin activity.

Serum-potassium has a striking action upon aldosterone secretion, which may rise several fold in response to changes of serum-potassium within the physiological range.[11] In normal circumstances the disposal of excess dietary potassium through tubular excretion may be an important function of aldosterone, whereas the problem of sodium depletion is not encountered under usual dietary conditions.

Catecholamines have also been implicated in the control of aldosterone secretion, since autonomic insufficiency is sometimes accompanied by deficient renin release and low aldosterone-secretion rates. Such patients may show a deficient postural rise in renin release and aldosterone secretion on standing, and a poor aldosterone response to sodium deficiency.[12]

In general, the demonstrable effects of A.C.T.H. and angiotensin II on aldosterone secretion appear to be permissive rather than specific. Although excessive angiotensin II production does seem to stimulate aldosterone secretion in certain disease states, the normal regulation of aldosterone by sodium balance requires the operation of a further humoral factor or electrolyte effect within the cells of the zona glomerulosa. The results of biosynthetic studies[11] indicate that A.C.T.H. and angiotensin II stimulate early stages of biosynthesis, promoting the conversion of cholesterol to pregnenolone by mitochondria. Sodium depletion has a striking effect on the biosynthetic steps between corticosterone and aldosterone, and potassium stimulates the preceding step between desoxycorticosterone (D.O.C.) and corticosterone (fig. 21).

Secretion and Transport of Adrenal Steroids

Daily secretion-rates of the major adrenal steroids in man are: cortisol, 15 mg.; 17-ketosteroids, 20 mg.; and aldosterone, 50–200 μg. according to sodium balance (table II). The corresponding plasma-levels for cortisol are 16 (A.M.) to 8 (P.M.) μg. per 100 ml. and for aldosterone, 3–15 ng. per 100 ml. (table III). Secretion-rates are estimated over 24 hours by measuring the degree of isotope dilution after administration of the labelled steroid and isolation of a specific urinary metabolite, or over shorter periods as the product of the prevailing blood-clearance rate and peripheral level of steroid. In healthy individuals, glucocorticoid secretion is mainly influenced by stress, and aldosterone secretion by sodium balance and pregnancy. Obesity is sometimes associated with a rise in glucocorticoid secretion, though the blood-level remains normal.

TABLE III—PLASMA LEVELS OF MAIN ADRENOCORTICAL HORMONES

Steroid	Plasma-level (per 100 ml.)	
	Total	Free
Cortisol	5–20μg.	1000 ng.
Corticosterone	1 μg.	100 ng.
Aldosterone	3–15 ng.	3 ng.
Dehydroepiandrosterone	65 μg.	65 μg.

Most steroid hormones circulate in specific or non-specific association with plasma-proteins. The two specific binding proteins are corticosteroid-binding globulin (C.B.G., transcortin) which binds cortisol, and sex-hormone-binding globulin (S.H.B.G., also called testosterone-œstradiol binding globulin) which transports œstradiol and testosterone. In each case, the binding process depends upon the configuration of the steroid—C.B.G. binds steroids with Δ^4 3-ketone and 20-ketone groups,[14] while S.H.B.G. binds steroids with a 17βOH group. The blood-levels of both binding proteins are increased during pregnancy and œstrogen treatment, and each has been used to establish competitive assays for measurement of steroid hormones in blood. These specific binding proteins possess high association constants and low capacity, whereas plasma albumin, the major nonspecific binding protein, has much lower affinity and very high capacity.[15]

Under normal circumstances, the steroids circulate in association with the specific binding proteins, and only a small quantity is free. Thus, when the total plasma-cortisol level is 20 μg. per 100 ml., the 95% binding to C.B.G. results in a free cortisol level of only 1 μg. per 100 ml., which represents the metabolically active glucocorticoid in the circulation. The bound steroid acts as a reservoir when free cortisol is removed from plasma; C.B.G. becomes saturated when plasma-cortisol rises above 20–25 μg. per 100 ml. For this reason, any rise in total plasma-cortisol above normal, as in A.C.T.H. stimulation and Cushing's syndrome, will cause a proportionately much greater rise in plasma-free-cortisol. Therefore, quite small rises in glucocorticoid secretion can lead to features of glucocorticoid excess when C.B.G. remains normal (e.g., Cushing's syndrome), while increased secretion accompanied by increased C.B.G. levels, as in pregnancy, does not exert a proportionate metabolic effect. Any rise in plasma-free-cortisol is accompanied by a rise in urine-free-cortisol, which is, therefore, a valuable index of elevated cortisol secretion.[16]

Metabolism

The major metabolites of steroid hormones are formed in the liver, kidney, and gut, and excreted in the urine. During metabolism, the ring structure remains intact, the steroid being inactivated by reduction of the double bond and ketone groups, and rendered water-soluble by conjugation to form derivatives such as glucuronides and sulphates.[17] Corticosteroids are excreted largely as tetrahydro forms coupled to glucuronide, D.H.A. as sulphate, progesterone as pregnanediol, testosterone as reduced compounds (androsterone and ætiocholanolone) which appear in the urine with the larger bulk of 17-ketosteroids secreted by the adrenal, and œstradiol as conjugated forms after hydroxylation to œstriol or oxidation to œstrone. In all cases, small amounts of "free" steroid are excreted in the urine, but, except for urinary cortisol, the most useful measurements of urinary steroid excretion are done on the metabolites which comprise the major excretory products of the various steroid hormones.

Measurements of Steroids in Plasma and Urine

Chemical procedures such as the Zimmerman reaction for 17-keto-steroids and the Porter-Silber reaction for 17-hydroxycorticosteroids are widely used for urinary measurements, but are not so satisfactory to assay blood-levels. For several years, the use of isotope-derivative methods, in which plasma steroids were converted to radioactive derivatives, commonly acetates, and counted to measure the steroid mass, were the most reliable and sensitive method of plasma-steroid assay.[18] Such methods are too complex for general use, and have been supplemented by a variety of simpler techniques for assay of the major steroid hormones. Gas-liquid chromatography has been widely applied to steroid measurement, but is not generally used due to limitations on sample numbers, though pregnanediol assay is readily performed by this method. Fluorimetric assay has been valuable for clinical estimation of plasma-cortisol, and protein-binding assays are becoming popular for a variety of plasma steroids, including cortisol, progesterone, testosterone, and œstradiol. These assays make use of the moderately specific plasma binding proteins to measure steroids by displacement of the tritium-labelled steroid from combination with the binding protein.[19] Such assays are essentially isotope-dilution procedures in which the binding protein provides a specific "biopsy" of the steroid mixture and measures the extent of dilution of radioactive steroid by added steroid. The technique has been applied to all of the major plasma steroids except aldosterone, for which isotope-derivative assay is still the standard method. Similar binding techniques have been introduced by the use of cell-receptor molecules to measure œstradiol and A.C.T.H., and antibodies to steroids have been used to provide rapid and sensitive assays for plasma œstradiol and aldosterone. For clinical purposes, the most useful measures of adrenal function are provided by the urinary corticosteroid excretion measured by chemical assay, and the plasma-cortisol measured by fluorimetric or binding assay.

Disorders of Adrenal Steroid Secretion

Adrenal Insufficiency

Adrenal insufficiency is most commonly due to unexplained atrophy of the adrenal cortex, sometimes associated with failure of other endocrine glands and often accompanied by the presence of circulating autoantibodies to adrenal tissue. The resulting deficiency of both mineralocorticoid and glucocorticoid secretion leads to sodium loss, hyperkalæmia, low blood-pressure, hypoglycæmia, and other features. Secretion of both A.C.T.H. and M.S.H. is excessive, causing the characteristic pigmentation of Addison's disease. The acute presentation as a shocked patient (addisonian crisis) requires immediate diagnosis and treatment with large doses of intravenous glucocorticoid (cortisol, not synthetic steroids), fluid replacement with glucose-saline, and antibiotic cover for possible precipitating infection. Proof of the diagnosis may have to be delayed until treatment has been given; a blood-sample taken before therapy will later show low plasma-cortisol levels compared to those found in other shocked patients with normal adrenal function. The more chronic form of adrenal insufficiency presents most commonly with weakness, postural hypotension, gastrointestinal upsets, and pigmentation. The diagnosis of primary adrenal insufficiency is confirmed by the finding of low plasma and urine steroids, which do not rise after treatment with A.C.T.H. Small responses may occur in occasional patients with partial adrenal atrophy, and in those with primary disturbance of A.C.T.H. release due to hypothalamic or pituitary disease leading to secondary adrenal atrophy. The latter group frequently retain adequate, but low, aldosterone secretion, do not usually present an addisonian picture, and may show the features of hypopituitarism, including pallor instead of pigmentation. Plasma-A.C.T.H. assays render the distinction very easily, being extremely high in primary adrenal failure and low in pituitary disease. Such assays are not yet widely available, and an indirect test of pituitary function has been used to make this distinction. When 11β-hydroxylation is inhibited selectively by metyrapone in healthy individuals, the formation of cortisol is prevented and 11-desoxycortisol is secreted instead. In healthy individuals, the decline in blood-cortisol causes increased A.C.T.H. release from the pituitary, thereby stimulating steroidogenesis in the blocked adrenal followed by secretion of large quantities of 11-desoxycortisol. The rise in plasma level of this steroid, and the resulting increase in urinary 17-hydroxycorticosteroid metabolites, can be used to assess the integrity of the feedback control system, and to detect hypothalamic or pituitary lesions[20] (fig. 23). More recently, the ability of the pituitary to secrete A.C.T.H. has been tested directly by A.C.T.H. assay,[21] and indirectly by the rise in plasma-cortisol which occurs during insulin-induced hypoglycæmia for simultaneous assessment of G.H. secretion. When primary adrenocortical failure is proven, replacement with cortisone and a salt-retaining synthetic steroid such as 9α-fluorocortisol is started, the cortisone being transiently increased during infections and other stress.

Cushing's Syndrome

Excessive secretion of adrenal steroids by hyperplastic and neo-

. plastic lesions of the adrenal cortex leads to the characteristic picture of Cushing's syndrome, with predominant manifestations of glucocorticoid excess. The classic features of moon face, regional obesity, hypertension, atrophic skin with striæ, atrophic connective tissue and bone matrix, and diabetic glucose tolerance, are identical with those seen in therapeutic steroid overdosage.

Cushing's syndrome is usually caused by steroid-secreting tumours of the adrenal cortex or by bilateral adrenal hyperplasia (fig. 23); sometimes the disease is associated with nodular adrenal hyperplasia, an intermediate condition between adrenal adenoma and hyperplasia.

Adrenal tumours are more common in women, and the more malignant forms are often associated with excess androgen production. The usual adrenal adenoma is characterised by autonomous secretion of cortisol, being relatively uninfluenced by suppression with dexamethasone or stimulation with A.C.T.H. The plasma-A.C.T.H. in such patients is suppressed to subnormal levels.

Adrenal hyperplasia usually results from excessive A.C.T.H. secretion from the pituitary. Though only 10% of these patients show a demonstrable pituitary lesion, the plasma level of A.C.T.H. is elevated to several times normal. The regulatory system for A.C.T.H. release seems to be set at an abnormally high level, so that the high plasma-cortisol does not exert negative feedback on the hypothalamus. The mechanism is still responsive to high levels of glucocorticoid, and inhibition of A.C.T.H. release and cortisol secretion usually occurs (>80%) when dexamethasone 8 mg. daily is given. The hyperplastic glands are also responsive to stimulation by administration of A.C.T.H. and metyrapone.

Adrenal hyperplasia due to A.C.T.H. production by various carcinomas, notably lung cancer, is becoming more frequently recognised. This "ectopic A.C.T.H. syndrome" follows release of A.C.T.H.-like peptides by the tumour cells,[22] and is unresponsive to dexamethasone suppression. Such patients do not present the usual cushingoid picture, but show muscle wasting and hypokalæmia due to extremely high secretion of cortisol and desoxycorticosterone by the hyperplastic adrenals. Plasma-A.C.T.H. levels are considerably higher than in adrenal hyperplasia caused by pituitary overactivity. These and other neoplasms of non-endocrine tissues, commonly of foregut origin during development, may secrete a variety of peptide hormones in addition to A.C.T.H.—M.S.H., parathyroid hormone, A.D.H., gastrin, glucagon, and gonadotrophin have been recognised.

It is interesting that the production of steroid hormones from a non-endocrine tumour has not yet been described.

Cushing's syndrome is usually easily diagnosed by measurement of blood and urine cortisol levels, and 17-hydroxycorticoid excretion. A useful screening test is based on the ability of 1 mg. dexamethasone to suppress the morning plasma-cortisol levels in normal subjects, but not in Cushing's syndrome. A consistent feature of Cushing's syndrome is loss of the normal diurnal variation of plasma-cortisol. In some patients, plasma levels are not abnormally high, but are maintained at the morning level throughout the day, leading to clinical features of glucocorticoid excess.

To distinguish between the causes of Cushing's syndrome, suppression and stimulation tests and radiological studies are essential. Normal cortisol secretion is suppressed by dexamethasone 2 mg. daily, while 8 mg. daily will usually suppress secretion from hyperplastic glands maintained by pituitary A.C.T.H. release. Adrenal tumours, nodular hyperplasia, and hyperplasia caused by ectopic A.C.T.H. production do not usually suppress at the higher dosage. Hyperplastic glands will respond to A.C.T.H. administration with even higher secretion of cortisol, and to metyrapone by a rise in desoxycortisol and urine steroid excretion; in the ectopic A.C.T.H. syndrome, the responses to A.C.T.H. and metyrapone are sometimes subnormal or absent. The pituitary-adrenal relationship in the various forms of adrenal hyperfunction are summarised in diagrammatic form in fig. 23.

Treatment of Cushing's syndrome due to adrenocortical adenoma is by surgical resection of the tumour, commonly necessitating unilateral adrenalectomy. Bilateral adrenal hyperplasia is most effectively treated by total adrenalectomy; when pituitary overactivity is responsible, various forms of pituitary ablation such as irradiation, yttrium implantation, and cryogenic lesions have been found useful in some cases. If a pituitary tumour is present, surgical hypophysectomy should be performed. A moderate number of patients (about 10%) develop A.C.T.H.-secreting pituitary tumours a few years after adrenalectomy for bilateral adrenal hyperplasia. These tumours cause notable pigmentation and eventual visual impairment, and, as with the tumours which sometimes accompany the onset of adrenal hyperplasia, are commonly of chromophobe nature and may become locally invasive.

Various chemical inhibitors of adrenal function have been used to

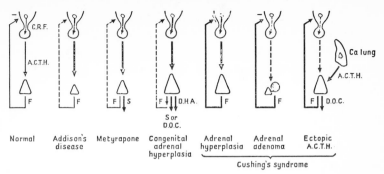

Fig. 23—Secretion of A.C.T.H. and corticosteroids in various disorders of adrenal function.
F = Cortisol. S = Desoxycortisol. D.H.A. — Dehydroepiandrosterone.
D.O.C. — Desoxycorticosterone.

reduce cortisol hypersecretion, most frequently in functioning carcinoma of the adrenal. Of these 1,1-dichloro-2-(o-chlorophenyl)-2-(p-chlorophenyl) ethane (o,p-D.D.D.) has been the most effective, and aminoglutethimide and metyrapone have also been used for selected cases. After surgical treatment of Cushing's syndrome, replacement therapy with cortisol is given as for other forms of adrenal insufficiency. Patients with adrenal hyperplasia require high initial replacement dosage, for several weeks, before reducing to the usual dose of about 30 mg. cortisone daily. After removal of an adrenal adenoma, smaller replacement dosage is required, sometimes for several months, until the atrophic contralateral adrenal has regained normal functio⁻

Hyperaldosteronism

Primary aldosteronism (Conn's syndrome) is usually produced by small single tumours of the adrenal cortex, though it may sometimes result from multiple tumours and rarely from hyperplasia of the zona glomerulosa. The classic clinical picture includes moderate hypertension, hypokalæmia, and the absence of œdema.[23] Sodium retention is present, but the renal escape mechanism permits normal sodium balance after an initial expansion of extracellular-fluid volume has occurred, while negative potassium balance is almost always present and progressive. The expanded plasma volume leads to suppression of renin secretion, and the combination of increased aldosterone secretion and suppressed plasma-renin level is highly suggestive of primary aldosteronism. Measurement of aldosterone-secretion rate and levels in urine and plasma are complex procedures, and various screening tests have been used to distinguish the rare cases with primary aldosteronism from the many who are investigated for the disorder, based on the plasma and urine potassium levels during sodium loading.[24] Aldosterone excretion is usually elevated, but may be normal in some patients, especially those with profound hypokalæmia. Sodium restriction and diuretics do not alter the aldosterone secretion nor elevate the suppressed plasma-renin, and sodium loading does not reduce aldosterone secretion. These features are usually sufficient to distinguish between primary aldosteronism and the secondary form which is sometimes associated with accelerated hypertension, renovascular hypertension, and other forms of renal disease. In particular, renin and angiotensin levels are high in all renal conditions causing secondary hyperaldosteronism, and plasma-sodium tends to be low rather than high.

In addition to the forms of secondary aldosteronism which accompany renal disease and hypertension, extremely high secretion-rates of aldosterone may occur in patients with cirrhosis and ascites, and the nephrotic syndrome. In these and other œdematous states, the kidney fails to escape from the effect of aldosterone, and sodium retention ensues, furthering the œdema and failing to suppress the stimulus for excess aldosterone secretion. Treatment of such patients with spironolactones, which block the action of aldosterone on the renal tubule, is often combined with diuretic therapy to achieve successful control of the œdema.

The existence of mild cases of aldosteronism with hypertension, normal serum-potassium, and, sometimes, normal but fixed aldosterone secretion has been demonstrated. The relationship of these few patients to the more usual picture is not yet clear, but there is no reason to believe that such subtle forms of aldosterone excess comprise more than a minute fraction of the general hypertensive population. A few rare cases have been described with A.C.T.H.-dependent hyperaldosteronism, the excessive secretion being suppressed by dexamethasone treatment.

The tumours which usually cause Conn's syndrome are rarely more than 3 cm. across, so preoperative localisation is not easy. Recently, cannulation of adrenal veins has been performed to allow preoperative estimations of aldosterone in order to localise the tumour, and retrograde adrenal angiography has been used. After resection of the tumour, transient relative hypoaldosteronism may lead to sodium loss and potassium retention, due to long-standing suppression of aldosterone secretion by the normal adrenal tissue. The hypertension usually subsides after surgery, but the persistence of high blood-pressure in certain cases seems to indicate that the adrenal lesion was not contributing to the hypertension, but merely accompanying it. Such patients usually have normal adrenals, or hyperplasia of the zona glomerulosa caused by an undetermined stimulus. The adenoma of Conn's syndrome is not totally autonomous, and may respond to angiotensin administration with a rise in aldosterone secretion. However, patients with aldosteronism are extremely sensitive to the pressor effects of angiotensin, and should not be given infusions of the peptide.

Congenital Adrenal Hyperplasia

Enzyme defects have been shown to occur at each of the major steps of corticosteroid biosynthesis from cholesterol, resulting in deficient formation of end-products such as cortisol, increased pituitary secretion of A.C.T.H., adrenal hyperplasia, and excessive androgen secretion. Accumulation of the immediate precursor at the site of block leads to varying degrees of masculinisation due to deviation into excessive androgen synthesis.[25]

21-hydroxylase deficiency is the commonest cause of congenital adrenal hyperplasia. Failure to hydroxylate the 21-carbon atom of progesterone causes accumulation of progesterone and 17-OH progesterone, leading to excess formation of androgens including testosterone. At the same time, synthesis of cortisol and aldosterone is blocked to varying degrees, causing limited glucocorticoid and mineralocorticoid secretion. In most cases, the urine excretion of 17-hydroxycorticosteroids is low or normal, and does not rise with further A.C.T.H. stimulation. A specific abnormality is the presence of large quantities of pregnanetriol, the metabolite of 17-OH progesterone, in urine.

About 50% of patients with 21-hydroxylase deficiency show striking sodium loss in early life, mainly due to inability to secrete adequate amounts of aldosterone. In some patients with the salt-losing syndrome, aldosterone secretion seems normal, and the formation of salt-losing steroid by the adrenal has been proposed. With advancing age, the electrolyte disturbance becomes less severe, and the major features are those of androgen excess and glucocorticoid deficiency. Treatment with cortisone suppresses the excessive A.C.T.H. secretion and corrects the abnormal steroid secretion. Plastic surgery is required in some children with severe genital deformity, but most are less severely affected and undergo relatively normal sexual development.

11β-hydroxylase deficiency is the second commonest variety of congenital adrenal hyperplasia, accounting for about 10% of cases. The degree of enzyme block may be variable, but the usual clinical features include virilisation and hypertension. The block of 11β-hydroxylation results in deficient synthesis of cortisol, leading to excessive A.C.T.H. release and adrenal hyperplasia, with elevated secretion of 11-desoxycortisol, D.O.C., and ketosteroids. The hypertension in this condition is due to the excessive D.O.C. secretion, and does not seem to be mediated only by sodium retention. The capacity to secrete aldosterone is limited, and salt depletion may occur in some infants with 11β-hydroxylase deficiency. With increasing age, D.O.C. secretion and sodium intake increase, eventually leading to sodium retention and hypertension. The steroid disturbances seen in patients with congenital adrenal hyperplasia caused by 11β-hydroxylase deficiency are similar to those which occur during administration of metyrapone and are corrected by replacement therapy with cortisone.

17-hydroxylase deficiency is extremely rare, and results in failure to form steroids derived from 17-hydroxylated precursors such as 17 OH-progesterone and 17 OH-pregnenolone.[26] This prevents synthesis of cortisol and sex hormones, since the enzyme deficiency occurs also in the gonad. The few patients recognised so far have been predominantly adult females, with absent secondary sexual features (due to œstrogen deficiency) and hypertension. The secretion of D.O.C. and corticosterone is increased by the greater availability of progesterone and the stimulation of A.C.T.H., leading to salt retention and hypertension, sometimes with hypokalæmia. Aldosterone secretion is usually low, possibly secondary to the sodium retention and depressed plasma-renin caused by the high D.O.C. secretion, and partly to an intra-adrenal action of the excess A.C.T.H. secretion in reducing aldosterone synthesis. Treatment of these patients with small doses of glucocorticoid suppresses the excessive A.C.T.H. release, reducing the excessive D.O.C. secretion and correcting the hypertension and hypokalæmia.

Other rare forms of congenital adrenal hyperplasia occur, but those described above are the usual variants of the disease. In all cases, correcting the cortisol deficiency by replacement therapy suppresses the excessive A.C.T.H. secretion and stops the channelling of large quantities of precursor molecules into other pathways leading to androgen synthesis (C21 and C11 defects) or corticosterone synthesis (C17 defect).

1. Ashmore, J., Weber, G. *in* Carbohydrate Metabolism and its Disorders (edited by F. Dickens, P. J. Randle, and W. J. Whelan); p. 335. New York, 1968.
2. Edelman, I. E. *in* Progress in Endocrinology (edited by C. Gual), p. 24. Amsterdam, 1969.
3. Grant, J. K. *J. Endocr.* 1968, **41**, 111.
4. Glenn, F., Peterson, R. E. Mannix, H. Surgery of the Adrenal Gland. New York, 1968.
5. Yates, F. E. *in* The Adrenal Cortex (edited by A. B. Eisenstein); p. 133. Boston, 1967.

6. Desaulles, P. A., Rittel, W. *in* The Investigation of Hypothalamic-Pituitary Adrenal Function (edited by V. H. T. James and J. Landon); p. 125. London, 1968.
7. Garren, L. D., Davis, W. W., Gill, G. N., Moses, H. L., Ney, R. L., Crocco, R. M. *in* Progress in Endocrinology (edited by C. Gual); p. 102. Amsterdam, 1969.
8. Newton, M. A., Laragh, J. H. *J. clin. Endocr. Metab.* 1968, **28**, 1006.
9. Davis, J. O. *in* The Adrenal Cortex (edited by A. B. Eisenstein); p. 203. Boston, 1967.
10. Pickering, G. High Blood Pressure; p. 102. London, 1968.
11. Blair-West, J. R., Cain, M., Catt, K., Coghlan, J. P., Denton, D. A., Funder, J. W., Scoggins, B. A., Wright, R. D. *in* Progress in Endocrinology (edited by C. Gual); p. 276. Amsterdam, 1969.
12. Gordon, R. D., Kuchel, O., Liddle, G. W., Island, D. *J. clin. Invest.* 1967, **46**, 599.
13. Burwell, L. R., Davis, W. W., Bartter, F. C. *Proc. R. Soc. Med.* 1969, **62**, 1254.
14. Daughaday, W. H. *in* The Adrenal Cortex (edited by A. B. Eisenstein); p. 385. Boston, 1967.
15. Rosner, W. *New Engl. J. Med.* 1969, **281**, 658.
16. Ross, E. J. *J. clin. Endocr. Metab.* 1960, **20**, 1360.
17. McKerns, K. W. Steroid Hormones and Metabolism. New York, 1969.
18. Kilman, B., Peterson, R. E. *J. biol. Chem.* 1960, **235**, 1639.
19. Murphy, B. E. P. *Rec. Prog. Hormone Res.* 1969, **25**, 563.
20. Liddle, G. W., Island, D., Meador, C. K. *ibid.* 1962, **18**, 125.
21. Berson, S. A., Yalow, R. S. *J. clin. Invest.* 1968, **47**, 2725.
22. Liddle, G. W., Nicholson, W. E., Island, D. P., Orth, D. N., Abe, K., Lowder, S. C. *Rec. Prog. Hormone Res.* 1969, **25**, 283.
23. Conn, J. W. *Harvey Lect.* 1968, **62**, 257.
24. Mulrow, P. J. *in* Diseases of Metabolism (edited by P. K. Bondy); p. 1083. Philadelphia, 1969.
25. Bongiovanni, A. M., Root, A. W. *New Eng. J. Med.* 1963, **268**, 1283, 1342, 1391.
26. Biglieri, E. G., Herron, M. A., Brust, N. *J. clin. Invest.* 1966, **45**, 1946.

CHAPTER SIX

The Thyroid Gland

THE thyroid gland synthesises and releases iodinated thyronine molecules which strongly influence metabolic processes and growth. The thyroid hormones are stored not in the gland cells as in other endocrine organs, but in colloid-containing vesicles enclosed by thyroid epithelium, as a precursor protein, thyroglobulin. Within the thyroglobulin molecule, tyrosine residues are iodinated to form monoiodotyrosine (M.I.T.) and diiodotyrosine (D.I.T.), which then combine to form the iodothyronines (fig. 24). The structural simi-

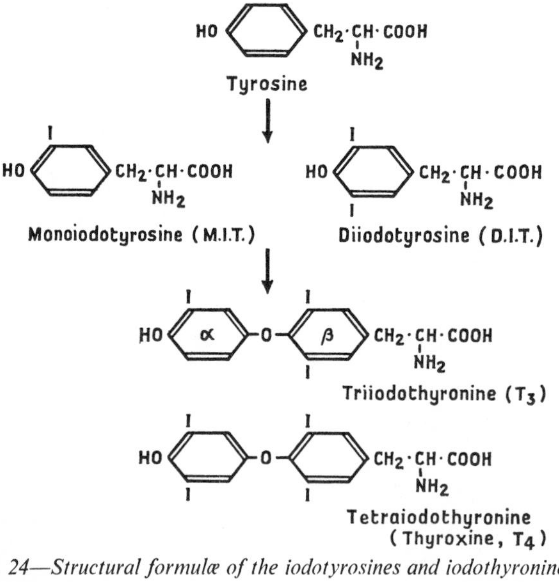

Fig. 24—*Structural formulæ of the iodotyrosines and iodothyronines.*

larity of the thyroid to an exocrine gland is due to its evolutionary origin from the endostyle, an organ which secretes iodinated mucoprotein into the pharynx of protochordata.[1] During vertebrate evolution, the thyroid has lost its functional and anatomical connection with the gastrointestinal tract and has developed as an endocrine organ of vital importance for metabolism and growth.

The thyroid hormones affect oxygen consumption and heat production in the whole animal and stimulate the metabolism of isolated tissues, particularly liver and muscle. The mechanism of this stimulation is not yet clear, but the hormones seem to act finally on the energy-producing electron-transfer processes in the respiratory enzyme systems of the mitochondria. Thyroid-hormone administration alters the number and physical structure of the mitochondria and reduces the efficiency of oxidative phosphorylation. These changes may be manifestations of excess hormone action; the effect of thyroid hormones at the physiological level involves increased transcription of messenger R.N.A., probably via cyclic A.M.P. The resulting increase of protein synthesis in mitochondria and microsomes is necessary for the subsequent stimulation of cell respiration caused by thyroid hormones. There is no single site of action which explains the multiple effects of thyroid hormones, which seem to act on the nucleus, endoplasmic reticulum, and mitochondria of responsive cells.[2] They also accelerate many other processes: protein breakdown is increased in collagen and other tissues, carbohydrate and lipid turnover are increased, calcium is mobilised from bone, and the heart-rate is accelerated. Several of the actions of thyroid hormone are consistent with increased sensitivity of β-receptors to catecholamines. In addition, an important action on body growth and maturation results from the direct effect of thyroxine on tissue growth and a permissive effect on growth-hormone secretion by the anterior pituitary gland.

All vertebrates have a follicular arrangement of thyroid tissue and produce similar thyroid hormones by iodination and degradation of thyroglobulin. In some species the thyroid hormones assume special functions—e.g., oxygen consumption in fish, metamorphosis in amphibia, and plumage growth in birds. Mammals have a general requirement for thyroid hormone in many aspects of metabolism and growth. In man, the thyroid develops as an outgrowth from the pharynx, in association with the parathyroids derived from the 3rd and 4th branchial arches and the ultimobranchial body from the 6th arch. The cells of the ultimobranchial body become incorporated within the developing thyroid gland, giving rise to the parafollicular or "C" cells, which are the source of calcitonin in mammals.[3] In lower vertebrates the ultimobranchial gland develops as a separate body below the parathyroids and contains a high concentration of calcitonin.

The initial development of the thyroid does not depend on trophic-hormone secretion from the pituitary; T.S.H. appears in the fetal pituitary at 11–12 weeks' gestation, corresponding to the time of active thyroid differentiation and colloid accumulation. Thereafter, T.S.H. is essential for continued development and regulation of thyroid function. The adult gland mass of 15–20 g. is maintained by the trophic action of pituitary T.S.H., the height of the follicular epithelial cells being related to the prevailing level of T.S.H. secretion. The trophic hormone also has a pronounced effect on the vascularity of the gland, comparable to the action of A.C.T.H. on the adrenal. Hypophysectomy causes complete atrophy of the thyroid gland, indicating the absolute dependence on T.S.H. secretion for maintenance of the normal structure. The opposite situation of thyroid overstimulation by excessive pituitary T.S.H. secretion is almost unknown; overproduction of glycoprotein hormones by the pituitary is extremely uncommon, and pituitary tumours producing thyrotrophin or gonadotrophins are exceedingly rare in man. Production of T.S.H.-like hormones by certain trophoblastic tumours has been recognised, sometimes leading to increased thyroid activity and mild clinical features of hyperthyroidism.

Iodine Metabolism[4]

Most dietary iodine is excreted in urine, within about 6 days of ingestion. Several other tissues share the thyroid's ability to concentrate iodide from plasma—notably the gastric, salivary, and mammary glands—but the thyroid has the most efficient trapping mechanism, accumulating up to 40 times the serum-level of iodide. Only the thyroid uptake is responsive to T.S.H., and only the thyroid incorporates iodine into iodothyronines. About 90% of body iodine is in the thyroid gland, mainly as organic iodide in thyroglobulin. This large pool of iodine (5000–7000 μg.) in the thyroid gland turns over very slowly, at about 1% daily.

The thyroid-follicle cells actively take up iodide against a substantial negative electrical gradient, and the accumulated iodide then diffuses rapidly into the follicular lumen. Organic binding of iodine also proceeds rapidly, and the capacity of the transport mechanism may be apparent only after blocking organification by inhibitors such as thiouracil. Other anions compete for iodide transport, and perchlorate or thiocyanate will stop iodine accumulation in the gland. If the thyroid contains a lot of inorganic iodide, as in certain biosynthetic defects, this unincorporated iodide will be discharged after perchlorate administration. The activity of the thyroid iodide trap is affected by T.S.H. and abnormal stimulating factors but not by thiouracil-type drugs. This trapping activity can be assessed in man by measuring the radioactivity over the thyroid gland 20 minutes after an intravenous dose of radioiodine or pertechnetate. The early uptake is normally below 8% of the administered dose and is substantially elevated in thyrotoxicosis.[5]

Radioiodine-uptake studies have previously been of importance in the diagnosis of thyroid disorders, but more direct measures of hormone-production rate are now more widely used. Radioiodine uptake by the gland can be used to evaluate iodide trapping at various times after administration of the isotope. Very early measurements, as described above, are not influenced by antithyroid drugs and can be used to evaluate thyroid function during treatment of thyrotoxicosis. Most commonly, the 24-hour uptake after an oral tracer dose of ^{131}I or ^{132}I is measured and is normally 15–20% of the administered dose. Much more clearcut separation between hypothyroid, normal, and thyrotoxic states can be obtained by the measurement of thyroid hormones in blood. It is likely that radioiodine-uptake studies will become reserved for special purposes, such as the assessment of thyroid trapping during antithyroid-drug treatment and the investigation of certain biosynthetic defects.

Thyroid-hormone Synthesis

The formation of thyroxine (T4) and triiodothyronine (T3) proceeds by a sequence of reactions which occur in the thyroglobulin molecule under the control of pituitary T.S.H. Thyroglobulin, a glycoprotein (M.W. 650,000) synthesised in the follicular cells and stored within the follicles as colloid, acts as a reservoir of thyroid hormones. Each 19S thyroglobulin molecule contains 115 tyrosine residues and consists of four 8S subunits which are iodinated during and after aggregation to form the complete molecule. The formation of thyroid hormones proceeds by the following stages:

1. *Iodination of tyrosyl residues to form M.I.T. and D.I.T.*—Oxidation of iodide to iodine by a peroxidase enzyme system is followed by spontaneous iodination of accessible tyrosine molecules in thyroglobulin. This is thought to take place at or near the surface of the thyroid follicle cells, leading to approximately equal numbers of M.I.T.

and D.I.T. residues in the iodinated thyroglobulin when iodine intake is normal.

2. *Coupling reaction between iodotyrosine residues.*—Suitably situated molecules of M.I.T. and D.I.T. undergo a coupling reaction to form T4 or T3. The nature of the coupling reaction is not clear, but possibly no enzyme system is involved. The steric relations between adjacent M.I.T. and D.I.T. residues are extremely important, and disruption of the tertiary structure of thyroglobulin modifies the rates of both iodination and coupling. At low levels of iodination, thyroxine formation is reduced when the thyroglobulin molecule is unfolded by guanidine; at high levels of iodination, T4 formation is enhanced, showing that D.I.T. residues can couple even when the polypeptide is in the random-coil form. Under normal conditions, coupling occurs readily between adjacent iodotyrosine residues on the surface of the thyroglobulin molecule.[6] In the rat, iodine deficiency is accompanied by a fall in the residues of D.I.T. and T4 per molecule of thyroglobulin, and a rise in M.I.T. and T3 formation. In man, iodine deficiency is also associated with a rise in the M.I.T./D.I.T. ratio and preferential production of T3, leading to a euthyroid state in the presence of a low protein-bound iodine (P.B.I.).

3. *Release of thyroid hormones from thyroglobulin.*—The epithelial follicular cells take up thyroglobulin colloid droplets by pinocytosis (fig. 25), and it is in these cells that thyroid hormones are released by degradation of thyroglobulin. In the cytoplasm, lysosomes coalesce with the droplets, releasing hydrolytic enzymes which degrade thyroglobulin to liberate thyroxine, triiodothyronine, M.I.T., and D.I.T. Deiodination of iodotyrosines takes place in the follicle cells, and the iodothyronines are secreted into the parafollicular capillaries along with minute quantities of thyroglobulin and iodotyrosine.

As well as thyroglobulin, the human thyroid gland forms albumin-like 4S iodoproteins which contain mainly M.I.T. or D.I.T. These may appear in the serum in certain thyroid disorders, and sometimes contribute to the P.B.I.

Thyroid-stimulating Hormone

Thyroid-stimulating hormone (thyrotrophin, T.S.H.) is a glycoprotein of M.W. 25,000 which is secreted by specific pituitary cells under the influence of a tripeptide releasing factor (T.S.H.R.F. or T.R.F.) formed in the hypothalamus and transported to the anterior pituitary via the portal vessels. The secretory granules (about 100 mμ diameter) in the thyrotrophin-secreting basophils take up glycoprotein stains. After thyroidectomy, these cells show marked hypertrophy, with increased endoplasmic reticulum and reduced granularity, reflecting the high rate of T.S.H. secretion. This hypertrophic response is caused by unopposed action of T.R.F. on the thyro-

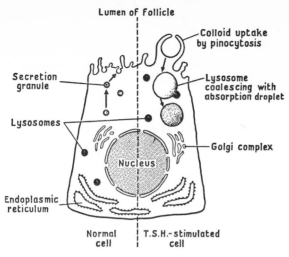

Fig. 25—Thyroid epithelial cell.

The left side shows secretory droplets being formed in the Golgi complex and discharged into the lumen of the follicle. The right side depicts the T.S.H. stimulated cell, showing colloid droplets being taken up by pinocytosis and coalescing with lysosomes. Degradation of thyroglobulin by hydrolytic enzymes is followed by release of thyroxine and triiodothyronine (from Fawcett et al.[21]).

trophs. Normally, thyroid hormones inhibit excessive T.R.F. action by a direct effect on the pituitary. T.R.F. has been isolated and characterised as a tripeptide with the structure (pyr)-glu-his-pro (NH_2), after years of research by Schally's[7] and Guillemin's[8] groups. This work involved the processing and fractionation of tons of sheep hypothalamus to yield a milligramme or so of purified material, for each hypothalamus contains only about a nanogramme of T.R.F. T.R.F. has been synthesised and shown to have full activity in man and other animals. It is active in vivo in nanogramme amounts and in vitro at the picogramme level, and it does not seem to be species-specific. T.R.F. causes a striking release of T.S.H. in vivo within seconds and is rapidly inactivated by plasma enzymes. The releasing effect of T.R.F. requires energy but does not involve protein synthesis; membrane depolarisation followed by Ca^{++} uptake has been proposed as the mechanism of activation of the storage granules. The effect of T.R.F. on the pituitary is inhibited by treatment with T4 or T3, which is consistent with the inhibitory feedback effect of thyroid hormones on T.S.H. secretion at the pituitary level. This inhibitory effect of thyroxine on T.R.F. action is mediated by a step involving protein synthesis (it is blocked by cycloheximide). The regulation of T.S.H. secretion by T.R.F. and T4 is shown in fig. 26. The hypothalamic release of T.R.F. may be relatively constant, except during acute exposure to cold. Otherwise, regulation occurs by interaction, at the thyrotroph cell, between T.R.F., thyroid hormone, and enzymes destroying T.R.F.[8] Enhanced peripheral utilisation of thyroid hormone leads to reduction of the feedback inhibition of T.R.F. action, resulting in further T.S.H. secretion and thyroxine formation to restore the blood-level to normal.

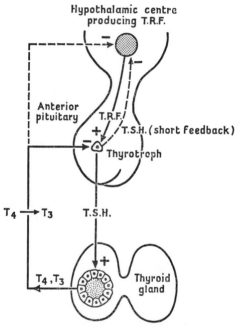

Fig. 26—Regulation of thyroid-hormone secretion.

Negative feedback by circulating thyroid hormone is exerted mainly upon the anterior pituitary, antagonising the driving action of T.R.F. on the thyrotrophin-secreting cells.

Actions of T.S.H. on the Thyroid

T.S.H. influences many aspects of thyroid structure and function: the size and vascularity of the gland, the height and activity of the follicular epithelium, and the amount of colloid are all controlled by

T.S.H. (fig. 25). Every step of the thyroid-hormone biosynthetic pathway is stimulated by T.S.H., as are numerous aspects of cell metabolism—e.g., glucose utilisation, oxygen consumption, phospholipid synthesis, and R.N.A. synthesis. These actions begin within a few minutes of administration of T.S.H. and have been attributed to activation of adenyl cyclase after combination with a receptor site on the cell surface.[9] The resulting formation of cyclic A.M.P. leads, via an effect on messenger R.N.A., to synthesis of proteins concerned in the individual steps of thyroid-hormone synthesis—i.e., the iodide trap, iodine incorporation into thyroglobulin, uptake and proteolysis of thyroglobulin, and thyroid-hormone release into the circulation.

Radioimmunoassay of Plasma-T.S.H.[10]

Radioimmunoassay methods have shown that T.S.H. secretion is normally constant after an initial rise and fall on the day of birth. Plasma-T.S.H. levels are raised in patients with primary hypothyroidism and undetectable in patients with hypothyroidism secondary to pituitary disease. In thyrotoxicosis, plasma-T.S.H. is almost always undetectable and never elevated, confirming the importance of abnormal stimulators or autonomous hyperfunction as the main factors in this disorder.

The elevated T.S.H. levels of hypothyroid patients are suppressed to normal by treatment with 200 μg. thyroxine daily for 7–21 days, or 100 μg. triiodothyronine daily for 3–10 days. In normal subjects T.S.H. levels are unresponsive to stimuli such as stress and cold, and even treatment with antithyroid drugs only occasionally produces a rise in plasma-T.S.H. Although T.S.H. is responsible for the development of most forms of non-toxic goitre, plasma-levels are elevated only in goitrous patients who have coexisting hypothyroidism. Euthyroid patients with multinodular goitre do not have elevated T.S.H. levels, though T.S.H. secretion was presumably increased during the development of the goitre. After treatment of thyrotoxicosis with radioiodine, persistent elevation of plasma-T.S.H. is sometimes seen in association with normal P.B.I. After treatment by subtotal thyroidectomy, the increase of T.S.H. declines after several weeks, as the thyroid remnant undergoes compensatory hypertrophy to a stage where adequate thyroid-hormone secretion occurs at normal T.S.H. levels. The radioiodine-treated gland seems unable to make the same growth response, and higher T.S.H. levels are necessary to maintain the same hormone output from the reduced gland mass.

Circulating Thyroid Hormone

The total amount of circulating hormonal iodine is 6–8 μg. per 100 ml. This is contained in thyroxine, with about 0.3 μg. per 100 ml. in triiodothyronine. Circulating thyroxine is strongly associated with plasma binding proteins, and the free plasma-hormone is less than 1/2000 of the total circulating level—i.e., only 3–4 ng. per 100 ml. The major binding proteins are thyroxine-binding globulin (T.B.G.), thyroxine-binding prealbumin (T.B.P.A.), and albumin, accounting for 60%, 30%, and 10% respectively of the thyroxine-binding capacity of plasma. The level of T.B.G. is influenced by œstrogen, and binding is increased during pregnancy and oral-contraceptive therapy. The triiodothyronine content of plasma is about 200 ng. per 100 ml.; T3 binds rather weakly to T.B.G. and is readily displaced by T4. Thyroxine was formerly believed to be the more important thyroid hormone, and many tests of thyroid function have been based on its measurement. The protein-bound iodine is largely thyroxine and correlates fairly well with thyroid activity, but it is affected by variations in T.B.G. level and iodinated contaminants in plasma. Total serum-thyroxine can be measured by displacement binding assay in a system including T.B.G. and labelled T4.[11] The saturation of the binding protein can be assessed by various in-vitro uptake tests, in which the uptake of labelled T3 to resin, charcoal, or red cells is used to provide a reflection of the free thyroxine in plasma. Less of the tracer T3 is bound by T.B.G. in the presence of high free-T4 levels, and therefore more radioactivity will be taken up by the adsorbent. This test is affected by pregnancy and œstrogen treatment, which increase the binding protein, causing a higher P.B.I. and decreased resin uptake. The best indirect estimate of free T4 is obtained by multiplying the P.B.I. or total serum-thyroxine by the T3 resin uptake to give the free-thyroxine index, which is more directly proportional to the true free-thyroxine level and eliminates the effects of variations in T.B.G.

Measurement of the serum-free-thyroxine by direct methods shows only about 3 ng. per 100 ml.; of the total serum-T3 (200 ng. per 100 ml.) about 1.5 ng. per 100 ml. is free. Despite the striking differences in total levels of these hormones, their free concentrations are relatively similar.

The biological activity of T3 is several times greater than that of T4, and the metabolic effects are more rapid. The metabolism of T3 is also more rapid, the turnover-rate being about 5 times that of T4. The daily secretion and utilisation of T4 is about 80 μg., and that of T3 is about 50 μg. There is increasing evidence that T3 may be as important as or more important than thyroxine in determining hormonal status.[12]

Metabolism of Thyroid Hormones

T.B.G. is probably important for the regulation of thyroid-hormone metabolism, by limiting the concentration of free hormone in the circulation. However, thyroxine turnover remains constant despite changes in plasma-binding. The exchangeable cellular thyroxine level has been supposed to determine thyroidal-hormone flux. Alteration in cellular binding and metabolism may operate through changes produced in the total exchangeable pool, affecting pituitary receptor cells.[13]

About 10% of the thyroxine secreted each day is excreted in the bile, mainly as free thyroxine and to some extent as the glucuronide. All hormone not eliminated in this way is metabolised by peripheral tissues and deiodinated, the iodide being excreted in the urine or recycled to the thyroid. The organic iodine in tissues is mainly thyroxine: whereas a proportion of T3 is present, there is no evidence that T4 is metabolised to T3 as the active form after entering cells. The major sites of thyroxine metabolism are liver and muscle. Inactivation of thyroid hormones proceeds by steps such as deiodination, oxidative deamination, and conjugation, all pathways being present in the liver. In the liver the site of metabolism is the smooth endoplasmic reticulum. The action of thyroxine seems to be accompanied by a specific deiodination of the α ring, followed by formation of an activated iodothyronine-protein complex with iodine confined to the β ring.[14]

Thyroxine undergoes substantial conversion to triiodothyronine after secretion, contributing up to 50% of the daily production of T3. Thus, thyroxine can act both directly on tissue metabolism and indirectly as a prohormone from which a more active component is formed.

Disorders of Thyroid Function

Excessive Thyroid-hormone Secretion

Hyperthyroidism occurs most frequently in Graves' disease (thyrotoxicosis, with associated goitre and exophthalmos) and in the autonomous hyperfunction of thyroid adenomas. Excessive secretion of thyroid hormones causes numerous clinical features related to increased metabolic activity and sensitivity to catecholamines. Nervousness, tremor, tachycardia, and goitre are almost always present, and sweating, heat intolerance, fatigue, weight-loss, increased vascularity of the gland, and eye signs are seen in the majority of patients. The secretion-rate of thyroid hormones is greatly increased, sometimes more than 10 times normal. The metabolic disposal of thyroid hormones is also increased, and the plasma-levels of thyroxine and triiodothyronine are elevated. Basal metabolic rate is almost always increased, the P.B.I. is above the normal upper limit of 8 μg. per 100 ml., the T3 resin uptake is increased because more T.B.G. binding sites than usual are occupied by thyroxine, and the serum-thyroxine itself is above the normal range. The mean serum-triiodothyronine is 3 to 4 times the normal value, being always well above the normal range of 170–270 ng. per 100 ml.[15] Cases of thyrotoxicosis have been observed with normal P.B.I. and serum-thyroxine and high levels of serum-triiodothyronine (400–1500 ng. per 100 ml.). Such examples of "T3 thyrotoxicosis" can occur in patients with nodular, diffuse, and recurrent toxic goitre. Other diagnostic features of thyrotoxicosis include a high radioiodine uptake by the gland and failure to suppress radioiodine uptake or P.B.I. by treatment with T3 for 2–3 weeks.

The pathogenesis of Graves' disease has been attributed to thyroid circulating abnormal stimulators with T.S.H.-like actions, leading to goitre and excessive thyroid-hormone secretion. The thyroid overactivity is independent of pituitary function—an autonomy which is reflected in the failure of T3 to suppress thyroid activity—and plasma-T.S.H. levels are low, owing to feedback from the excess thyroid-hormone secretion. Using a bioassay for plasma-T.S.H. based on the release of thyroidal radioactivity in animals pretreated with ^{131}I, Adams[16] detected a long-acting thyroid stimulator (L.A.T.S.) in the plasma of patients with thyrotoxicosis. This stimulator characteristically has a slower and more sustained effect than T.S.H., giving a

maximum bioassay response at 16 hours, instead of the 3 hours with
T.S.H. L.A.T.S. can be detected in the serum of most thyrotoxic patients,
at levels which correlate more closely with orbital disease and pre-
tibial myxœdema than with the severity of hyperthyroidism. The
identification of L.A.T.S. as a γ-globulin produced by lymphocytes of
patients with thyrotoxicosis suggests that it may be an autoantibody
to a thyroid antigen.[17] Adsorption of L.A.T.S. by homogenates prepared from human thyroid tissue has been demonstrated, and occurs
primarily in the endoplasmic reticulum of the microsomes. The
separated heavy chain of the L.A.T.S. molecule has short-acting
thyroid-stimulating activity, while recombination of the chains
restores the original long-acting stimulation. L.A.T.S. activity is neu-
tralised by antiserum to human γ-globulin but not by antiserum to
T.S.H., though the mechanism of action of L.A.T.S. on the thyroid
appears similar to that of T.S.H. Stimulation of organ function by an
autoantibody is not usual but could result from antibody formation
to a thyroid component with a regulatory function in thyroid-hormone synthesis.

The ability of thyroid tissue to inactivate T.S.H. is shared by
thymus and lymphatic tissue. The frequent enlargement of thymus and
lymph-nodes in Graves' disease may be related to this ability to
metabolise T.S.H. and to abnormal production of antibody with a
configuration similar to that of the active site of T.S.H. Demonstration that regression of Graves' disease has followed removal of the
enlarged thymus supports the possibility that thymic and lymphoid
cells may form L.A.T.S.

L.A.T.S. biological activity has been transferred experimentally to
human recipients, and transplacental passage of L.A.T.S. seems to be
the cause of neonatal hyperthyroidism in infants of thyrotoxic
mothers. Nevertheless, the presence of L.A.T.S. does not alone provide
an adequate explanation for all aspects of Graves' disease—the
levels in serum do not correlate well with thyroid size, and the rapid
appearance of thyroid suppressibility in some patients after antithyroid-drug treatment is not consistent with the relatively long half-
life of L.A.T.S. (about 18 days).

In patients with hyperfunctioning thyroid adenoma, eye signs and
muscle weakness do not occur, and L.A.T.S. activity is not detectable
in the serum. Localised uptake of radioiodine by the adenoma can
often be demonstrated, and the serum P.B.I. and T4 are elevated.
Toxic multinodular goitre usually occurs as a complication of non-

toxic nodular goitre, with relatively mild hyperthyroid features and often normal radioiodine uptake and P.B.I. The suggestion that some patients may be secreting T3 rather than T4 is strengthened by the finding that many patients with non-toxic nodular goitre show slight elevation of serum-T3.[18]

Thyrotoxicosis can be controlled by blocking thyroid-hormone secretion with antithyroid drugs, or by ablation of the hyperactive gland by surgery or radioiodine. Measures directed at suppression of abnormal stimulators are also beginning to be applied. In general, it is easy to make patients euthyroid, but all methods have disadvantages, and management must be carefully designed for each patient. Treatment with iodine alone causes rapid but transient improvement by blocking the release of thyroid hormone, and it has been widely used during preparation for surgery. Antithyroid drugs such as propylthiouracil and carbimazole ('Neo-Mercazole') block thyroid-hormone synthesis by inhibiting the coupling of iodotyrosines and by acting upon a sulphonyl-iodide intermediate in the iodination of tyrosine. About 50% of patients are cured during a course of antithyroid-drug treatment for a year. Ablative treatment of thyrotoxicosis is more effective and rapid, but in about 40% of patients it is followed eventually by the development of hypothydroidism. Hypothyroidism seems to be the only complication of radioiodine therapy, whereas surgery, which is followed less often by hypothyroidism, has other complications, such as hypoparathyroidism and damage to the recurrent laryngeal nerves. Attempts have been made to improve the results of treatment by combining antithyroid drugs with reduced doses of radioiodine. One such approach, involving treatment with half the usual ^{131}I dose followed by antithyroid-drug treatment for up to 2 years, has substantially reduced the 5-year incidence of hypothyroidism.[19] Another approach uses serial 20-minute radioiodine-uptake measurements to assess the suppressibility of the thyroid iodide trap during treatment with antithyroid drugs and T3, to detect unresponsive patients who are more suitable for treatment with radioiodine or surgery.[5]

For treatment of toxic multinodular goitre, larger doses of radioiodine are given during temporary cessation of antithyroid-drug therapy. Such patients are often elderly and have associated heart-disease, and surgery is used only for obstructive symptoms. When toxic adenoma is present, surgical excision is preferable to radioiodine treatment.

To achieve a rapid symptomatic remission in thyrotoxicosis, treatment with a β-adrenergic blocking agent (propranolol) has been used before treatment with antithyroid drugs, radioiodine, or surgery. In this way the tachycardia and nervousness can be controlled within a week, facilitating the use of more slowly acting definitive methods of treatment.

Deficient Thyroid-hormone Secretion

Hypothyroidism may result from atrophy or loss of thyroid tissue or from biochemical disorders of thyroid-hormone synthesis which cause compensatory oversecretion of T.S.H. and goitre formation. In each case, the peripheral effects of thyroid-hormone deficiency are apparent. Decreased metabolism, bradycardia, cold sensitivity, skin thickening by mucinous œdema, intellectual deterioration, mental and physical lethargy, and slow hoarse speech are commonly seen. Physical examination usually reveals striking delay in relaxation of tendon reflexes. Primary hypothyroidism is much commoner in women than in men and is often associated with the presence of circulating thyroid autoantibodies. Serum-T.S.H. levels are always raised, and serum thyroxine and T3 are below normal. The P.B.I. is usually low, and treatment with T.S.H. does not stimulate thyroid-hormone secretion. In pituitary hypothyroidism, skin changes are less noticeable, and other features of hypopituitarism may be present. Plasma-T.S.H. is undetectable, the low P.B.I. responds to treatment with bovine T.S.H. for 3 days, and the plasma-growth-hormone response to hypoglycæmia is defective. Hypothyroidism is treated with thyroxine replacement and can be monitored if necessary by the P.B.I., though the clinical response is usually an adequate guide. Replacement by T3 does not raise the P.B.I. and is particularly indicated for treatment of myxœdema coma, owing to its faster action than thyroxine.

Various defects in thyroid-hormone synthesis lead, through increased T.S.H. secretion, to compensatory hypertrophy of the thyroid. In some cases, such as the endemic goitre of iodine deficiency, this compensation results in a euthyroid state; although the P.B.I. is often low, most patients are not hypothyroid, owing to preferential formation of T3. Genetic factors play some part in determining the efficiency of adaptation to iodine deficiency, for only a proportion of susceptible individuals develop goitre. Endemic cretinism usually occurs in children of goitrous parents; the slow mental development and growth retardation of infantile hypothyroidism are often accompanied in endemic cretinism by neurological disturbances caused by thyroid-hormone deficiency during early fetal life. Although iodine deficiency is not the sole factor in the development of endemic goitre and endemic cretinism, these conditions are almost eliminated by programmes which ensure adequate intake of iodine in the diet.

Sporadic goitrous cretinism is usually due to an inherited defect of thyroid-hormone biosynthesis.[20] At least six metabolic defects may lead to goitre and hypothyroidism; these include an iodide-trapping defect, inability to incorporate iodine into thyroglobulin, failure of iodotyrosine coupling, defective deiodination of M.I.T. and D.I.T., and impaired proteolysis of thyroglobulin. Treatment with thyroid hormone must be instituted early in all forms of cretinism to avoid permanent effects on mental development and growth.

1. Means, J. H., DeGroot, L. J., Stanbury, J. B. *in* The Thyroid and its Diseases; chap. 1. New York, 1963.
2. Rawson, R. W., Money, W. L., Greif, R. L. *in* Diseases of Metabolism (edited by P. K. Bondy); p. 768. Philadelphia, 1969.
3. Pearse, A. G. E., Carvalheira, A. F. *Nature. Lond.* 1967, **214**, 929.
4. Wayne, E. J., Koutras, D. A., Alexander, W. D. Clinical Aspects of Iodine Metabolism. Oxford, 1964.
5. Alexander, W. D., Harden, R. McG., Shimmins, J. *Rec. Prog. Horm. Res.* 1969, **25**, 423.
6. Edelhoch, H. Progress in Endocrinology (edited by C. Gual); p. 415. Amsterdam, 1969.
7. Nair, R. M. G., Barrett, J. F., Bowers, C. Y., Schally, A. V. *Biochemistry*, 1970, **9**, 1103.
8. Guillemin, R., Burgus, R., Vale, W. *in* Progress in Endocrinology (edited by C. Gual); p. 577. Amsterdam, 1969.
9. Pastan, I. *ibid.* p. 98.
10. Utiger, R. D. *in* Progress in Endocrinology (edited by C. Gual); p. 1186. Amsterdam, 1969.
11. Murphy, B. E. P. *Rec. Prog. Horm. Res.* 1969, **25**, 563.
12. Sterling, K. *ibid.* p. 415.
13. Oppenheimer, J. H., Surks, M. I., Schwartz, H. L. *ibid.* p. 381.
14. Galton, V. A. *in* Recent Advances in Endocrinology (edited by V. H. T. James); p. 181. Boston, 1968.
15. Sterling, K., Bellabarba, D., Newman, E. S., Brenner, M. A. *J. clin. Invest.* 1969, **48**, 1150.
16. Adams, D. D. *J. clin. Endocr.* 1958, **18**, 699.
17. McKenzie, J. M. *Physiol. Rev.* 1968, **48**, 252.

18. Bellabarba, D., Séguin, P. *Clin. Res.* 1970, **18**, 355.
19. Smith, R. N., Wilson, B. M. *Br. med. J.* 1967, i, 129.
20. Stanbury, J. B., Wyngaarden, J. B., Fredrickson, D. S. Metabolic Basic of Inherited Disease; p. 215. New York, 1966.
21. Fawcett, D. W., Long, J. A., Jones, A. L. *Rec. Prog. Horm. Res.* 1969, **25**, 315.

CHAPTER SEVEN

Hormonal Control of Calcium Homœostasis

SERUM-CALCIUM is normally maintained within narrow limits by homœostatic mechanisms which regulate the two roles of calcium—its mechanical function in bone, and the metabolic actions of ionised calcium on cell-membrane permeability, neuromuscular activity, blood coagulation, and enzymic and secretory processes. Plasma-calcium fluctuates daily within $\pm 3\%$ regardless of calcium intake and excretion, and acutely induced changes in serum-calcium are quickly restored to normal. This regulation involves the integrated actions of parathyroid hormone ("parathormone"), calcitonin, and vitamin D in controlling calcium absorption, bone turnover, and excretion of calcium and phosphorus.

McLean[1] postulated that calcium homœostasis involved two processes—a physicochemical exchange of calcium between bone and plasma, and a hormonal (parathyroid) mechanism to maintain the blood-level above that created by the exchange process. The skeleton contains a large reservoir of calcium in the form of tiny bone crystals, which provide a vast area for mineral exchange. About 1% of the total body-calcium is present in the circulation and soft tissues, and a further 1% of the skeletal calcium is available for free exchange. The skeleton is in a continuous state of metabolic turnover, calcium being deposited at sites of bone formation and released in other areas by bone resorption. This turnover is high in young animals and declines with age. In the absence of hormonal controls, exchangeable bone mineral acts as a crude buffer of the serum-calcium level, which is maintained around 6 mg. per 100 ml. instead of the usual range of 9·0–10·4 mg. per 100 ml. To maintain and regulate the normal range of serum-calcium, endocrine tissues derived embryologically from the branchial arches secrete parathormone and calcitonin, which act on bone respectively to raise and lower the serum-calcium level. In addition, parathormone acts on kidney and gut to regulate plasma-calcium by controlling the excretion and absorption of calcium. In normal circumstances, these actions may be more important in calcium regulation than the effect of parathormone on bone.

Parathormone[2]

The parathyroids respond to hypocalcæmia by secreting parathormone, a single-chain polypeptide of 83 aminoacid residues (M.W. 8500) with biological activity in the N-terminal half of the molecule. Parathormone is not stored in the parathyroid glands but is synthesised and secreted continuously; since no storage granules are present and the tissue content is extremely low, the isolation of parathormone has been difficult.

The action of parathormone in bone is twofold—an early effect on osteocytes leading to calcium release from mature bone crystals into blood, and a slower effect on bone turnover and remodelling during maintained hypersecretion. The early effect occurs within 15–30 minutes and does not initially depend on R.N.A. synthesis by the osteocytes. Parathormone also acts directly on the kidney to reduce calcium clearance and enhance phosphate excretion, and on the gut to increase calcium absorption. The actions of parathormone on bone and kidney have been shown to involve stimulation of adenyl cyclase and increased formation of cyclic A.M.P., and cyclic A.M.P. has been found to increase calcium resorption and release into blood.[3]

The secretion of parathormone has been studied by radioimmunoassays utilising antibodies to the bovine hormone. Such studies have shown that serum-parathormone concentration is inversely related to serum-calcium, falling to zero when the serum-calcium exceeds 12 mg. per 100 ml. (fig. 27). Secretion is stimulated when serum-calcium is lowered by edetic-acid infusion, and is strikingly increased during lactation[4]; the hormone is rapidly cleared from the circulation with a half-life of 18 minutes.

In man, blood-parathormone assays are difficult; serum-levels are often undetectable in normal subjects but are usually elevated in patients with primary or secondary hyperparathyroidism. In renal failure, altered metabolism of parathyroid hormone has been observed during radioimmunoassay studies.

Calcitonin

In 1961, Copp[5] recognised a further hormonal control of calcium homœostasis in the form of a hypocalcæmic factor which he termed "calcitonin". This became apparent when perfusion of dog thyroparathyroid glands with blood of high calcium concentration caused the systemic blood-calcium level to fall more rapidly than could be achieved by surgical thyroparathyroidectomy. Also, cautery of the parathyroids in the rat led to a faster fall of blood-calcium than did surgical excision of the glands from the subjacent thyroid glands.

Subsequent work showed that calcitonin was formed in the thyroid gland and not the parathyroids, the rapid hypocalcæmic effect of cautery in the rat being due to release of the hypocalcæmic factor following damage to the thyroid gland. Calcitonin is formed in mammalian thyroid parafollicular cells, which contain secretory granules of calcitonin that vary in abundance according to the blood-calcium level. These cells arise in fetal life from the ultimobranchial body, which develops from the last branchial arch and in mammals fuses with the thyroid gland. Calcitonin has also been identified in other mammalian tissues, including thymus and adrenal, but seems to arise predominantly in the thyroid. In other vertebrates the ultimobranchial gland develops as a body separate from the thyroid, and in birds, fish, and amphibia it contains high concentrations of calcitonin. The isolation and sequence analysis of human, porcine, bovine, and salmon calcitonin have been done, and the human, porcine, and salmon forms have been synthesised.

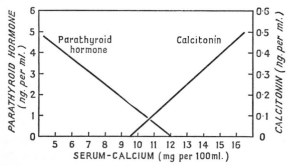

Fig. 27—Effect of serum-calcium changes on the levels of parathormone and calcitonin in peripheral blood.
Modified from Potts and Deftos.[2]

In all species, calcitonin is a linear peptide of 32 aminoacid residues (M.W. 3600); bovine and porcine calcitonin are similar, while the human hormone shows more numerous differences in structure.[2] Fish calcitonin is much more potent than the porcine and human hormones, and may be the most useful form of calcitonin for therapeutic purposes.

Radioimmunoassay and bioassay studies have shown that calcitonin is secreted continuously in normal animals, with elevations during hypercalcæmia and cessation of secretion during hypocalcæmia.[6] Secretion of calcitonin is directly proportional to blood-calcium, above the level of about 9 mg. per 100 ml.; below this level, the blood-calcitonin concentration is undetectable (fig. 27). The half-life of calcitonin in the circulation is shorter than that of parathormone, being only 4–12 minutes.[7]

The hypocalcæmic action of calcitonin is due to inhibition of bone resorption and calcium release. Bone catabolism is significantly reduced, and prolonged treatment causes an increase in trabecular-bone formation. Because the hypocalcæmic action depends upon bone resorption, this effect of calcitonin is more noticeable in young animals with rapid bone turnover. The mechanism of action of calcitonin on bone-cells does not seem to require R.N.A. or protein synthesis, nor to involve the adenyl-cyclase system. The exact function of calcitonin in the mammal has not yet been completely defined. It may be valuable primarily during periods of calcium stress, as in rapid bone growth in young animals, pregnancy and lactation, and egg-laying in birds. Calcium homœostasis in mammals seems to be controlled mainly by parathormone, with calcitonin as an accessory regulator during acute episodes of hypercalcæmia or as a fine adjustment under normal conditions (fig. 28). Copp[8] has compared the roles of parathormone and calcitonin in calcium regulation with those formerly attributed to insulin and glucagon in glucose homœostasis.

Vitamin D

Since 1953, vitamin D has been recognised as being essential for the action of parathormone on bone, as well as for the absorption of calcium in the gut. Dietary vitamin D is converted to an active metabolite by hydroxylation at the 25 position by a hepatic enzyme system.[9] The active form of vitamin D localises in the cell nucleus and influences the transcription of messenger R.N.A. in intestine and bone, leading to formation of calcium-transport systems in these tissues. In bone, the transport protein induced by vitamin D may operate as shown in fig. 29, in conjunction with parathormone and calcitonin. In the acute sense, parathormone enhances the permeability of the cells to calcium, and calcitonin has the opposite effect.[10] However, parathormone also has a more prolonged effect on bone resorption,

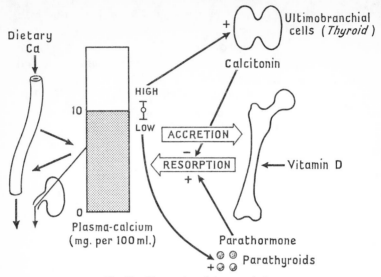

Fig. 28—Factors in calcium regulation.

Parathormone also has important actions on calcium regulation by the kidney and gut. From Copp.[5]

involving new R.N.A. synthesis by osteocytes and breakdown of bone matrix with release of hydroxyproline. Calcitonin opposes the initial action of parathormone on calcium release but not the more prolonged effect on bone resorption. Vitamin D is essential for the hypercalcæmic action of parathormone but not for the hypocalcæmic action of calcitonin. The active 25-hydroxylated form of vitamin D may well be regarded as a hormone secreted by the liver into the circulation after formation from an inactive precursor.[10] Like other steroid hormones, it stimulates the formation of specific messenger R.N.A. within the nucleus of its target tissues.

Disorders of Parathyroid Secretion

Hyperparathyroidism

Parathormone secretion is increased in primary hyperparathyroidism due to adenoma or hyperplasia of the parathyroids and in hyperparathyroidism secondary to chronic renal disease or associated with osteomalacia. In longstanding secondary parathyroid overactivity and hyperplasia, autonomous parathyroid function sometimes develops and has been termed tertiary hyperparathyroidism.

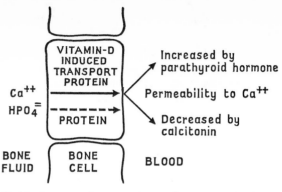

Fig. 29—Model of actions of vitamin D, parathormone, and calcitonin on bone mobilisation.

Vitamin-D-induced protein in bone-cell aids transport of calcium from bone-fluid to bone-cell. Parathormone increases permeability to Ca^{++}, calcitonin decreases it. (After DeLuca.[10])

Primary hyperparathyroidism most commonly presents with renal calculi or gastrointestinal symptoms, and rarely with bone disease. Serum-calcium is elevated, but sometimes only slightly above normal, and serum-alkaline-phosphatase is often normal. Precise measurement of serum-calcium is essential for accurate diagnosis and selection of patients for surgical treatment.

Definitive diagnosis may be difficult in some patients, and radio-immunoassay of serum-parathormone can be valuable in confirming the diagnosis.[11] The assay is not yet widely performed and has not been perfected, but it has shown that patients with primary hyper-parathyroidism generally have elevated plasma-levels of immunore-active parathormone. This is particularly apparent in relation to their prevailing high levels of serum-calcium. In patients with parathyroid hyperplasia, calcium infusion lowers the plasma-parathormone level and may provide a means for distinguishing between hyperplasia and the autonomous secretion of parathyroid adenomas and ectopic sources of parathormone. Treatment of primary hyperparathyroidism by surgical excision is sometimes complicated by difficulty in localising the glands, and various techniques have been used to overcome this problem. Preoperative catheterisation and radioimmunoassay of parathormone levels in the major veins draining the neck and thorax has been found useful in localising parathyroid adenomas in the neck and mediastinum. Also, assay of blood-parathormone levels after

massage of the neck has been used to determine the sites of parathyroid adenomas.[11]

Excess parathormone secretion may also occur from a variety of
malignant tumours, especially those arising in the lungs and kidney.
Such tumours may secrete peptides which are immunologically and
biologically similar to parathormone and can produce the same
clinical picture as primary hyperparathyroidism.

Hypoparathyroidism

This occurs most commonly after thyroid surgery and is less often
due to idiopathic atrophy of the parathyroids (which is sometimes
accompanied by evidence of an autoimmune disorder). Pseudohypo-
parathyroidism, a rare familial condition, shows all the features of
hypoparathyroidism but is caused by an end-organ resistance to
parathormone, which is secreted in excessive amounts. Cyclic-A.M.P.
formation in response to parathormone is deficient, indicating a defect
in the membrane-receptor/adenyl-cyclase system in responsive tissues
such as kidney and bone.

All forms of hypoparathyroidism need treatment to raise serum-
calcium to normal, since uncontrolled hypocalcæmia leads to
numerous pathological sequelæ, as well as characteristic neuromuscular disturbances (tetany and convulsions). Vitamin-D therapy
usually corrects the blood-calcium level effectively but is sometimes
difficult to control. Purified dihydrotachysterol is more effective but
more expensive; the active 25-hydroxylated form of vitamin D may
also provide more satisfactory therapeutic control than calciferol
itself.

Calcitonin Secretion

Disorders of calcitonin secretion in human bone disease have not
been detected, but high levels of calcitonin are present in the plasma
of patients with medullary carcinoma of the thyroid, which arises
from the parafollicular cells. Strangely, such patients do not become
hypocalcæmic, and the function of calcitonin in man has been ques-
tioned for this reason. It is possible that calcium homœostasis is
being maintained in these patients by increased parathyroid activity,
producing normal blood-calcium levels despite increased calcitonin
secretion. However, the absence of hypercalcæmia after thyroidectomy also casts doubt on the magnitude of the effect of calcitonin on
blood-calcium under usual conditions. Possibly its function is rela-

tively minor in man compared with other species, in which dietary calcium may show wide variations and calcium balance may fluctuate considerably during egg formation and lactation.[8]

Therapeutic uses for calcitonin have lately been suggested[12]: already acute hypercalcæmia has been successfully treated with calcitonin, and beneficial effects have been claimed in osteoporosis and Paget's disease.

1. McLean, F. C. *Clin. Orthop.* 1957, **9**, 46.
2. Potts, J. T., Deftos, L. J. *in* Diseases of Metabolism (edited by P. K. Bondy); p. 904. Philaelphia, 1969.
3. Chase, L. *Ann intern. Med.* 1969, **70**, 1243.
4. Potts, J. T., Buckle, R. M., Sherwood, L. M., Ramberg, F. C., Mayer, C. P., Kronfield, D. S. Deftos, L. J., Care, A. D., Aurbach, G. D. *in* Parathyroid Hormone and Thyrocalcitonin (Calcitonin) (edited by R. V. Talmage and L. F. Belanger); p. 407. Amsterdam, 1968.
5. Copp, D. H. *ibid.* p. 25.
6. Care, A. D., Leggate, J., O'Riordan, J. L. H., West, T. *in* Progress in Endocrinology (edited by C. Gual); p. 1181. Amsterdam, 1969.
7. Lee, M. R., Deftos, L. J. Potts, J. T. *Endocrinology*, 1969, **84**, 36.
8. Copp, D. H., Parkes, C. O. *in* Progress in Endocrinology (edited by C. Gual); p. 704. Amsterdam, 1969.
9. Blunt, J. W., DeLuca, H. F., Schoes, H. K. *Biochemistry*, 1968, **7**, 3317.
10. DeLuca, H. F. *in* Calcitonin 1969. Proceedings of the Second International Symposium; p. 205. London, 1970.
11. Reiss, E., Canterbury, M. S. *New Engl. J. Med.* 1969, **280**, 1381.
12. Foster, G. V., Clarke, M. B., Doyle, F. H., Joplin, G. F., Singer, F. R., Fraser, T. R., MacIntyre, I. *in* Parathyroid Hormone and Thyrocalcitonin (Calcitonin) (edited by R. V. Talmage and L. F. Belanger); p. 100. Amsterdam, 1968.

CHAPTER EIGHT

Insulin and Glucose Homœostasis

THE digestive functions of the gut depend upon the formation and activation of digestive enzymes under the control of local gastrointestinal hormones such as gastrin, secretin, and pancreozymin. The ensuing absorption of hydrolysed dietary constituents is accompanied by a further set of hormonal activities leading to cellular utilisation of small molecules for energy storage and synthetic processes. Normal eating habits provide intermittent loads of protein, carbohydrate, and fat in varying proportions; the hormonal events following absorption stimulate cellular uptake of sugar, aminoacids, and lipid, with utilisation for energy, conversion to larger storage molecules such as glycogen or fat, and synthesis of molecules concerned with cell structure and function. The major hormonal regulator of these metabolic processes is insulin, which interacts with growth hormone (G.H.), glucocorticoids, and catecholamines to promote nutrient storage and synthetic processes, and to regulate energy supply to tissues. After feeding, plasma-levels of glucose, aminoacids, and chylomicrons rise sharply, then return to normal as insulin increases their peripheral utilisation and storage. The adipose-tissue cells provide most of the daily energy requirements as free fatty acids (F.F.A.), especially during the intervals between feeding; only the brain, renal medulla, and red blood-cells have no alternative to glucose as an energy source. The dependence of these vital tissues on glucose metabolism requires that an adequate blood-sugar level is always available, and glucostatic mechanisms operate to maintain the blood-sugar above 60 mg. per 100 ml. during fasting by modulating glucose secretion from the liver.

During fasting, the glycogen stores rapidly become depleted, so that protein and fat must supply all energy needs after the first few hours; insulin secretion is reduced, favouring F.F.A. release from adipose tissue and reducing peripheral glucose utilisation. G.H. has been proposed to function as a hormone of fasting by causing F.F.A. release and reducing peripheral glucose utilisation, but catecholamines are probably more important factors in lipolysis. Glucocorticoids play an important part by promoting gluconeogenesis from protein, to provide the glucose necessary for metabolism by the specialised tissues. During prolonged fasting, cerebral metabolism shows partial adaptation to the utilisation of ketone bodies; after several days, glucose production from protein falls to about 20 g. daily, and adipose tissue provides about 95% of the total energy requirement.[1]

After feeding, insulin secretion is stimulated by several mechanisms; both glucose and aminoacids have direct effects upon insulin secretion, while further stimulation is provided by the gut hormones secreted during digestion and absorption.

The hormones regulating exocrine pancreatic function are important components of the physiological control of the endocrine function of the pancreas; they enhance the insulin response to glucose and aminoacids, and thus stimulate the peripheral utilisation of metabolic fuels.

Insulin is formed and stored in the β cells of the islets of Langerhans, which arise in the embryo from ducts originating from the gut and hepatic diverticula, and develop into highly vascular units of about 200 μ diameter. In man, the predominant cell type is the insulin-secreting β cell, which comprises 60–90% of the islet cells; a cells, which secrete glucagon, and gastrin-secreting D cells are also present in small numbers. The pancreas contains one to two million islets, representing a total mass of about 1 g. of tissue. Insulin is prepared from pancreatic tissue by steps including acid-ethanol extraction and zinc precipitation; the most purified material has a biological activity of 24 U per mg. The average insulin content of the pancreas is 200 U (8 mg.) and the daily secretion-rate is about 50 U (2 mg.), much of which is metabolised in the liver.

The insulin molecule is a small protein (M.W. 6000) composed of two peptide chains united by disulphide bonds (fig. 30). The A chain has 21 aminoacid residues, and the B chain 30 residues; aminoacid sequences differ between species, and some animals (fish and rodents) produce multiple forms of insulin. However, beef and pig insulin are similar to human insulin in all but a few residues, with three differences in the bovine molecule and only one in pig insulin. This similarity of structure is responsible for the relatively low antigenicity of the beef and pig insulins used for treatment of diabetes mellitus. Most insulin-treated diabetics develop low levels of antibody to the exogenous insulin, but rarely of sufficient titre to neutralise significant amounts of the insulin administered for treatment.

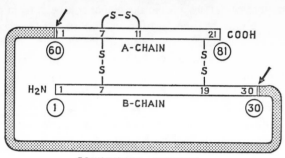

Fig. 30—Structure of proinsulin as determined by Steiner et al.[2]

The two-chain insulin molecule is formed by cleavage of proinsulin by a trypsin-like enzyme at the sites indicated by arrows, releasing the connecting peptide (shaded).

Insulin is a moderately insoluble protein, and polymerises in acid solutions. It also forms insoluble fibrils quite readily, and aggregation is favoured by the presence of zinc. The insulin molecule has been synthesised, but the scale of production is not yet sufficient to replace preparation from the pancreas of stockyard animals.

Insulin Biosynthesis

The formation of insulin in the β cell follows the usual pattern of polypeptide synthesis on the ribosome, under the control of triplet nucleotide sequences of mR.N.A. The characteristic two-chain structure of insulin is produced by partial proteolysis of a larger precursor molecule termed proinsulin.[2] The primary structure of the 84-aminoacid proinsulin chain causes the molecule to adopt a characteristic tertiary configuration, with formation of disulphide bridges which stabilise the molecule. A large connecting peptide (C-peptide) of 33 aminoacid residues is then selectively excised from the proinsulin molecule after cleavage at basic residues by a trypsin-like enzyme, leaving the two chains of insulin connected by disulphide bonds (fig. 30).

Proinsulin was first detected during incubation of islet-cell-tumour tissue with labelled aminoacids, and has since been found in plasma and urine and in many insulin preparations. It is released from the β cells in small amounts when insulin is secreted, and seems to be identical with the "big insulin" detected in plasma by gel filtration.[3] During biosynthetic studies, proinsulin is formed rapidly from aminoacids and converted into insulin with a half-time of one hour, consistent with the transit-time of proteins from ribosomes to secretory granules. The proteolytic cleavage of proinsulin is performed by trypsin-like enzymes within membranes of the Golgi apparatus or secretion granules, leaving only a small proportion of unconverted proinsulin, less than 5% of the pancreatic insulin content. The C-peptide formed during conversion of proinsulin to insulin is stored in the secretory granules and secreted along with insulin into the circulation.

Proinsulin has very low biological activity but shows 50% of the immunological potency of insulin by radioimmunoassay; therefore it can be detected by insulin radioimmunoassay systems after extraction from pancreatic tissue and plasma. In contrast, insulin shows little or no cross-reaction with antibodies against purified proinsulin. The antigenic activity of proinsulin is determined mainly by the C-peptide region of the molecule; since the C-peptide differs quite strikingly between species, immunoassays based on the bovine and porcine proinsulin are of little value in man. A radioimmunoassay for the human C-peptide has been developed to permit study of the release of proinsulin and the C-peptide in clinical disorders of insulin secretion.

In evolutionary origin, proinsulin may have been a digestive enzyme, cleaved by other proteolytic enzymes in the gut to liberate insulin which was absorbed into the bloodstream and reacted with cell membranes to stimulate the uptake of sugar, aminoacids, and lipid. The pancreatic β cell could have evolved from an intestinal cell responsible for synthesis of proinsulin, eventually secreting insulin directly into the bloodstream in response to other gut hormones, besides glucose and aminoacids.[2]

Secretion of Insulin

Insulin is secreted by the β cells in response to a variety of stimuli, including metabolic fuels, several peptide hormones, and certain autonomic transmitters.

After proinsulin synthesis and its conversion to insulin, the β cell seems to form two pools of insulin—a storage pool which responds to various stimuli by acute insulin release, and another pool which maintains the storage pool and provides the insulin secreted under basal conditions and during prolonged stimulation.[4] Many stimuli cause a brief initial burst of insulin secretion from preformed stores, followed by a more slowly rising level of secretion during maintained stimulation. This pattern is clearly seen during in-vitro stimulation of insulin release by glucose, which is the main physiological regulator of insulin secretion. Glucose causes a rapid release of insulin within 1 minute, rising to a peak at 2 minutes, and falling again to lower levels; this initial pulse is followed by a further rise beginning some minutes later and rising to high sustained levels at 30–60 minutes. The second phase is inhibited by puromycin, and probably reflects secretion of newly synthesised insulin.[5] The synthetic and secretory mechanisms of the β cell are separate, since some stimuli cause release of insulin from storage granules without increasing the rate of insulin synthesis. Glucose has a central role in β-cell function, promoting both the synthesis and secretion of insulin. Insulin synthesis depends largely upon glucose as an energy source, and proceeds at a rate proportional to the prevailing glucose concentration. G.H. also increases insulin synthesis by islet cells, but not the basal secretion of insulin; the insulin response to glucose is enhanced by G.H. treatment and in acromegaly.

Insulin secretion also responds directly to changes in glucose concentration; during in-vitro studies insulin release rises strikingly as the glucose level is increased from 100 to 500 mg. per 100 ml.[6] The β cell is fully permeable to glucose, which acts on secretion after being converted to glucose-6-phosphate and metabolised to produce A.T.P. The rate of glucose metabolism may be controlled by the intracellular level of cyclic A.M.P.; the β cell contains an adenyl-cyclase system which has been shown to enhance insulin secretion in the presence of glucose after activation by hormones (glucagon, A.C.T.H.) or β-adrenergic stimuli. Similarly, phosphodiesterase inhibitors such as xanthines, which raise the intracellular level of cyclic A.M.P. by preventing its breakdown to A.M.P., also increase the glucose-induced secretion of insulin.

Certain aminoacids directly increase insulin secretion when plasma-levels are elevated by infusion or ingestion, and have a synergistic effect with glucose on stimulating insulin release from the pancreas. Insulin increases aminoacid uptake and protein synthesis in muscle and adipose tissue, acting in unison with G.H.

Autonomic factors certainly participate in insulin secretion, to some extent via effects on the adenyl-cyclase system of the β cell. Adrenaline inhibits the glucose-induced stimulation of insulin release by blocking the early rapid phase of insulin release, an action mediated by an α-adrenergic mechanism which may act to reduce cyclic A.M.P. formation. (The effect of oral glucose is not inhibited, nor the actions of other factors which stimulate the more slowly responding intracellular pool to release insulin.) By contrast, β-adrenergic stimuli increase insulin secretion, and β-blocking agents inhibit it. Basal insulin secretion is increased by vagal stimulation and reduced by vagotomy, which does not alter the glucose effect on insulin release.

Besides the direct actions of glucose and aminoacids, hormones released from the gastrointestinal tract during absorption provide further stimuli to insulin secretion.[7] Glucose taken by mouth causes a much larger and more prolonged insulin response than when given intravenously, despite the lower plasma-glucose levels which follow oral glucose.[8] The enhanced insulin secretion during absorption of glucose and aminoacids causes these molecules to be more rapidly and effectively utilised than when given intravenously. All of the known gastrointestinal hormones stimulate insulin release from the islet cells – gastrin, secretin, and pancreozymin, as well as glucagon and a related peptide secreted by intestinal mucosa (gut glucagon[8,10] [fig. 31]). The functional significance of these actions during the physiological mechanisms accompanying digestion has not yet been established. Pharmacological effects of gastrointestinal factors on insulin release may result from minor chemical similarities between the various peptides, as may the immunological cross-reactions which influence the specificity of radioimmunossays for the gut hormones.

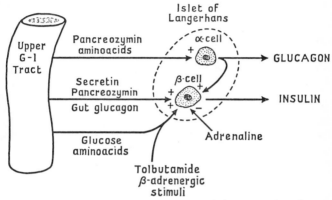

Fig. 31—Factors affecting the secretion of glucagon and insulin.

Despite these complications, there is increasing evidence that secretin may play an important role in augmenting the insulin response to glucose absorption and that pancreozymin may have a similar action during aminoacid absorption. Plasma-levels of secretin rise rapidly after glucose and protein ingestion; these responses are suppressed by insulin administration. Also, secretin levels are high in untreated diabetes and are reduced by insulin therapy, suggesting that feedback normally occurs between insulin and secretin.[11,12] The chain of gut hormones released during digestion (gastrin, secretin, and pancreozymin) may act synergistically to enhance and prolong the insulin response to absorbed glucose and aminoacids. The role of gut glucagon remains controversial; its secretion is stimulated during absorption of sugars, but does not reach a peak until the insulin response to glucose has subsided. Furthermore, the insulin-releasing effects of gut glucagon have yet to be confirmed using a highly purified preparation.

Pancreatic glucagon is a potent stimulus to insulin release, probably acting via the adenyl-cyclase system. It is normally a less effective stimulus than glucose; its action is not affected by adrenaline, so it may be important only when the normal glucose stimulus is inhibited by excessive levels of catecholamines or other factors. The hyperglycæmic response to glucagon follows the rise in plasma-insulin, so is not responsible for this action. Pancreatic glucagon secretion is reduced by oral glucose, in contrast to that of gut glucagon, and is stimulated by pancreozymin and aminoacids, and by hypoglycæmia. We do not yet know the extent to which the classic cyclic-A.M.P.-mediated glycogenolytic effect of glucagon operates to raise blood-glucose in normal circumstances.

Insulin secretion can also be stimulated by sulphonylurea compounds; tolbutamide and chlorpropamide are typical of these agents, which cause degranulation of β cells and a rapid rise in plasma-insulin. The hypoglycæmic action of sulphonylureas has led to their widespread use for the treatment of mild diabetes mellitus, especially for obese middle-aged patients with no tendency to ketoacidosis. Such patients have responsive β cells but are secreting insulin at a rate which is inadequate for their metabolic requirements. These oral hypoglycæmic agents have not been useful for the control of juvenile-onset diabetics, in whom deficient insulin secretion and β-cell failure are common. The insulin-releasing effects of tolbutamide are of diagnostic value in detecting insulin-secreting islet-cell tumours; intravenous administration of tolbutamide causes rapid and excessive insulin release from the islet-cell adenoma, followed by a more striking and prolonged fall of blood-sugar than in healthy individuals. The test can also be used to distinguish normal and diabetic patterns of insulin secretion, but is not necessary for the diagnosis of diabetes mellitus.

Insulin circulates in plasma at levels of about 20 μU per ml. plasma, rising after glucose ingestion to 50–150 μU per ml. The measurement of insulin by various forms of bioassay was complicated by the occurrence of plasma factors with insulin-like activity; since radioimmunoassay was introduced by Yalow and Berson,[13] the immunoreactive plasma-insulin has become established as the most valid measure of circulating insulin. Insulin does not circulate in association with plasma-protein, but as a monomer which is rapidly metabolised by liver and kidneys with a half-life of about 5 minutes. Small amounts of insulin are detectable in urine by radioimmunoassay, but measurement of plasma-insulin is most frequently used to give an estimate of insulin secretion and metabolism. Proinsulin contributes to the level of immunoreactive plasma-insulin, but is usually less than 20% of the total except in patients with islet-cell tumour of the pancreas.

Actions of Insulin

The biological effects of insulin are mainly concerned with nutrient storage and metabolism, and with anabolic processes. The best-known action is reduction of blood-sugar, due to enhanced glucose uptake in peripheral tissues and reduced hepatic output of glucose. In addition, insulin has extensive effects on metabolism, stimulating the synthesis of macromolecules involved in cell growth and function, promoting carbohydrate utilisation, and regulating energy production, storage, and release. Thus, insulin stimulates synthesis of glycogen in muscle and liver, of lipid in adipose tissue and liver, and of protein, R.N.A., and D.N.A. in cells generally. There is no single action of insulin which accounts for these diverse effects; the primary site of action is the cell membrane, with local effects on transport systems for sugar and aminoacids, and widespread activation of intracellular effector systems within sites such as genes and ribosomes. Although the formation of a common intracellular mediator such as cyclic A.M.P. could account for many of these multiple effects in various tissues, there is no evidence for such an action. Cyclic-A.M.P. formation is reduced by insulin in liver and adipose tissue, contributing to the antilipolytic action of insulin in these tissues. However, cyclic A.M.P. does not act as a positive mediator of insulin activity, in contrast to its major role in the action of hormones such as glucagon, A.C.T.H., and adrenaline, which exert actions on carbohydrate metabolism that are generally opposite to those of insulin.

Major sites of insulin action are the liver, adipose tissue, and muscle, the primary event being interaction with cell-membrance receptors. Prominent localisation of insulin at muscle and fat-cell membranes has been shown, and polymer-coupled insulin retains activity despite its inability to enter cells. The liver directly receives most of the insulin secreted by the β cells, and inactivates up to 40% of the hormone in a single passage. At the same time, insulin acts upon hepatic enzyme systems, stimulating those concerned with glycogen synthesis and glycolysis, and suppressing enzyme systems involved in gluconeogenesis. In adipose tissue, glucose uptake and conversion to fatty acids is enhanced by insulin, release of F.F.A. is inhibited, and fat synthesis is increased. The absence of insulin activity, as in fasting and diabetes, leads to enhanced lipolysis in adipose tissue via increased formation of cyclic A.M.P., with breakdown of fat stores to fatty acids and glycerol. Since adipose tissue cannot phosphorylate and reutilise the glycerol released during lipolysis, it diffuses from the fat-cells and is metabolised in the liver. The fatty acids released during insulin lack are metabolised to produce energy in muscle and liver; although the synthesis of fatty acids in the liver is inhibited by insulin lack, the supply of glycerol and fatty acid from peripheral fat depots leads to increased triglyceride synthesis in the liver during insulin deficiency. In muscle, the uptake of aminoacids and synthesis of protein are strongly stimulated by insulin, especially in younger animals. In the absence of insulin, glycolysis is reduced and glucose utilisation by muscle is impaired. In addition, insulin influences the function of muscle ribosomes, which show reduced ability to synthesise protein during insulin deficiency. Insulin may induce the formation of a specific regulatory protein which is necessary for ribosomes to function effectively in response to mR.N.A.

Insulin Antagonists

Although various non-hormonal insulin antagonists have been postulated on the basis of earlier bioassay studies, there are conflicting data about the validity of these factors, and little evidence of their physiological or clinical relevance. Hormones such as G.H., cortisol (hydrocortisone), pancreatic glucagon, and catecholamines are often described as physiological insulin antagonists, but exert multiple actions, including those which are opposite to the effects of insulin, to maintain glucose supply to the brain, to correct hypoglycæmia, and to provide F.F.A. for muscle metabolism.

G.H. administration acutely decreases the blood-levels of sugar and F.F.A., and is rapidly followed by an increase of plasma-F.F.A. and, after several hours, by decreased glucose tolerance. The early insulin-like effects may not represent physiological actions of G.H., and even the lipolytic action may not be a major physiological effect despite its attractiveness as a role of G.H. in the adult. Acromegaly is not usually accompanied by disturbed lipid metabolism, despite high G.H. secretion. The effect of G.H. on lipolysis may be largely synergistic with the actions of other lipolytic factors such as adrenaline, A.C.T.H., and insulin lack. However, there is no doubt that G.H. has physiological effects on carbohydrate metabolism and insulin secretion, mainly through decreased peripheral glucose utilisation.[14] G.H. inhibits glucose uptake by fat and muscle cells, leading to further insulin secretion which prevents a significant rise of blood-sugar. G.H. also enhances the islet-cell response to glucose, and glucose output from the liver. The overall effect of G.H. is to cause a compensatory oversecretion of insulin which maintains normal carbohydrate metabolism if pancreatic reserve is adequate. Certain species regularly develop hyperglycæmia after G.H. administration; in man, this happens only when high doses are given and pancreatic reserve is impaired. However, glucose tolerance is notably impaired several hours after a single injection of H.G.H., despite an accompanying rise in the glucose-induced secretion of insulin. In acromegaly, the excessive secretion of G.H. results in a combination of insulin resistance and increased capacity to secrete insulin; glucose tolerance is frequently abnormal, and about 25% of patients have overt diabetes mellitus. It seems likely that the diabetic syndrome develops only in those acromegalic patients with genetic predisposition to diabetes. Acromegalic patients without diabetes show a rapid and exaggerated rise of insulin secretion after glucose ingestion, arginine infusion, or tolbutamide administration; those with severely impaired glucose tolerance show the delayed insulin response characteristic of diabetic and prediabetic subjects. In G.H. deficiency, the insulin response to glucose ingestion is reduced, sensitivity to administered insulin is increased, due to lack of peripheral antagonism by G.H., and the recovery from insulin-induced hypoglycæmia is delayed.

Corticosteroids increase the availability of glucose precursors to the liver by promoting protein catabolism, and enhance the activity of the hepatic gluconeogenic enzyme systems. There is also an inhibiting action on peripheral glucose utilisation, and a synergistic effect on lipolysis in adipose tissue.

Adrenaline can activate hepatic and muscle glycogenolytic enzymes, increasing hepatic glucose output and enhancing gluconeogenesis from lactate. The secretion of adrenaline is increased by profound hypoglycæmia, but probably not by physiological variation in blood-sugar levels. Adrenaline also inhibits insulin secretion by the islet cells, and decreases glucose uptake by peripheral tissues. Although doubts have been expressed about the physiological relevance of these actions of adrenaline, when compared with the blood-levels of catecholamines, the local secretion of adrenaline from adrenergic nerve terminals to adjacent receptors may be a significant factor in glucose homœostasis. During fasting, increased catecholamine secretion contributes to fatty-acid mobilisation from adipose tissue, and also to the impaired insulin response to glucose which accompanies the carbohydrate intolerance of fasting.

Glucagon

Glucagon is a small peptide synthesised by the α cells of the islets of Langerhans, and released in response to hypoglycæmia and fasting. The hormone has a dramatic action on glucose production from glycogen in the liver, via formation of cyclic A.M.P. and activation of hepatic phosphorylase. These actions led to the view that glucagon is a hormone of glucose need, acting to repair acute falls in blood-sugar. This may be so in certain birds and reptiles, which show severe hypoglycæmia after pancreatectomy. However, glucagon is also a powerful stimulus to insulin secretion in man, and the understanding of its rcle in glucose regulation has been complicated by the presence of glucagon-like peptides released from intestinal mucosa during glucose absorption. This gut glucagon cross-reacts in the glucagon immunoassay, and has been proposed to act as an insulinogenic factor during absorption of food.[10] The relative roles of gut glucagon and pancreatic glucagon in glucose metabolism and insulin secretion have not yet been resolved. Purified pancreatic glucagon causes insulin release followed by hyperglycæmia when administered to healthy individuals. Endogenous pancreatic glucagon may function as a mediator of insulin secretion by local action within the islet upon adjacent β cells, after secretion in response to stimuli from the gut.[10]

Glucose Tolerance and Insulin Secretion

The blood-glucose time curve after 100 g. glucose taken by mouth is the simplest way to identify patients with abnormal carbohydrate tolerance. The most severe form of carbohydrate intolerance occurs in overt diabetes mellitus, and may be accompanied by a diagnostic elevation of the fasting blood-sugar above 120 mg. per ml. In healthy individuals, the fasting blood-glucose is 65–100 mg. per 100 ml.; after 100 g. glucose, the blood-glucose rarely rises above 180 mg. per 100 ml., and returns to normal in 2–3 hours. Diabetes mellitus causes an abnormally high fasting level, an excessive rise after oral glucose, and a delayed return to the normal level. Smaller deviations from the normal pattern of blood-glucose indicate the presence of "chemical diabetes," which may be a manifestation of early diabetes mellitus, or of other hormonal disorders.[j]

The measurement of plasma-insulin levels during the glucose-tolerance test gives much additional information about carbohydrate metabolism. In healthy individuals, glucose ingestion causes a rapid rise of insulin secretion with striking variation in the individual plasma responses. Obese subjects show elevated basal plasma-insulin values, and secrete two to four times as much insulin as normal after glucose ingestion. Obesity is associated with insulin resistance, and with compensatory hypersecretion of insulin; like acromegaly and pregnancy, obesity leads to diabetes when associated with impaired insulin secretory capacity.

Diabetes Mellitus

The syndrome of hyperglycæmia, glycosuria, and ketosis can result from several basic disorders which cause carbohydrate intolerance associated with features of relative or absolute insulin deficiency. Excessive secretion of hormonal antagonists can cause the diabetic syndrome, as in acromegaly, Cushing's syndrome, and phæochromocytoma, by reducing the effectiveness of insulin. Removal or destruction of the islets by surgery or pancreatitis produces more obvious features of insulin deficiency. Besides carbohydrate disturbances, these include protein catabolism and ketoacidosis accompanied by varying degrees of fluid and electrolyte depletion, progressing in severe cases to coma and death.

The usual form of diabetes mellitus is characterised by a genetically determined abnormality of insulin secretion. During glucose-tolerance tests, the plasma-insulin responds more slowly than usual, and may rise to reach and exceed the normal peak value in patients with mild diabetes. Obese diabetics show excessive insulin release compared with normal individuals, but secrete less insulin than the non-diabetic obese and usually show a delay in reaching peak values. Patients with severe diabetes often show absolute deficiency of insulin secretion with a delayed and attenuated response to glucose (fig. 32) .

Abnormal insulin secretion is detectable even in patients with minor glucose intolerance, and sometimes in subjects with prediabetes (i.e., those with a strong family history of diabetes). Despite the excessive insulin response found in mild and obese diabetics, the ratio of blood-glucose to plasma-insulin is usually subnormal. The exaggerated plasma-insulin response in these individuals represents a compensation to an underlying relative insensitivity to endogenous insulin. This resistance could be due to synthesis of insulin with impaired biological activity, or to interference with the action of insulin on its receptor sites. In all patients with diabetes mellitus there exists a relative or absolute deficiency of *insulin activity*, even

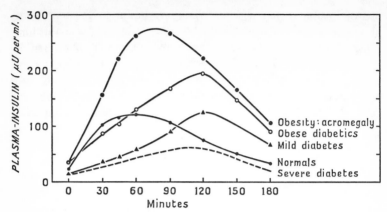

Fig. 32—Plasma-insulin responses to oral glucose (100 g.) in normal, obese, acromegalic, and diabetic individuals.

Compared to normals, acromegalic and obese subjects show marked hyper-secretion of insulin; in diabetes, the plasma-insulin response is slow, with a delayed peak which may exceed the normal response, especially in mild and obese diabetics.

though, in mild and obese diabetics, carbohydrate intolerance may be minimal and plasma-insulin can eventually rise to supranormal levels. Obesity is commonly associated with maturity-onset diabetes, and contributes to the insulin resistance and relative insulin deficiency in such patients.

In the severe juvenile-onset form of diabetes, the clinical disorder seems to develop very rapidly, with severe features of insulin deficiency and undetectable plasma-insulin. In fact, such children often pass rapidly through the same phases as adult diabetics, with chemical diabetes, prediabetes, and subclinical diabetes preceding the appearance of overt diabetes.

The inheritance pattern of diabetes has not been clarified, though there is clearly a strong genetic factor influencing the development of the disease. Dietary factors also play a major part in determining the incidence of diabetes; obesity is commonly associated with maturity-onset diabetes, and contributes to the insulin resistance and relative insulin deficiency of such patients, in whom dietary restriction is of primary importance in controlling the manifestations of diabetes.

The disturbance of pancreatic endocrine function is not accompanied by consistent pathological changes in the islet cells. The β cells are often reduced in numbers, especially in juvenile-onset diabetes, and show varying degrees of hyaline degeneration in diabetes of long duration. There is no conclusive evidence about the chemical nature of diabetic insulin, though some studies have detected altered resistance of plasma-insulin to enzymic and physical attack. Whether abnormalities of the proinsulin/insulin conversion can occur has not yet been determined; genetically determined defects in the connecting peptide sequence could affect the molecular configuration of proinsulin and limit the capacity of the β cells to form and secrete insulin.[2]

The widespread vascular complications of diabetes include non-specific atheromatous changes in large vessels and characteristic abnormalities of basement membranes in small vessels. Besides the typical lesions in renal glomeruli and retinal vessels, pronounced basement membrane thickening has been found in muscle capillaries of diabetes and in a high proportion of the children of diabetic parents.[15]

Such changes have not been found in patients with other forms of hyperglycæmia, and may represent a primary lesion of the diabetic process. The disturbance of capillary basement-membrane structure may lead to impairment of insulin efficacy and release, and to disturbed carbohydrate tolerance as secondary manifestations of the disease.

Management of Diabetes

Despite the possibility that abnormal carbohydrate metabolism could be a secondary feature of diabetes, control of the blood-sugar is still regarded as the first aim of therapy. Such control will certainly reduce the risk of diabetic ketoacidosis, and may lessen the incidence and severity of long-term complications such as diabetic retinopathy. Dietary management is directed at attaining normal weight, and providing adequate caloric intake according to individual needs. While many mature-age obese diabetics are controlled by diet alone, the juvenile-onset form and some adult-onset diabetics require insulin for correction of their abnormal metabolic pattern, and to avoid the development of ketoacidosis. Oral hypoglycæmic agents have been widely used for treatment of mild diabetes in middle-aged patients, and act by stimulating the β cells to secrete more insulin (sulphonylurea compounds) or by augmenting the action of insulin on muscle (diguanides). However, the results of long-term studies have indicated that the effectiveness of oral hypoglycæmic therapy for diabetes may not be superior to treatment by diet alone. Furthermore, it has been claimed that the death-rate from cardiovascular disease in tolbutamide-treated diabetics is more than twice that for treatment with diet or diet plus insulin.[16] If this is so, it would obviously be appropriate to place more emphasis on reduction of the adipose-tissue mass of maturity-onset diabetics and less on the augmentation of insulin secretion by drug therapy.

Patients requiring insulin treatment for control of diabetes are usually first put on small doses of long-acting insulin plus an appropriate diet. In patients with more severe diabetes and a tendency to acidosis, frequent smaller doses of short-acting insulin are given during the first few days, followed by a change to a longer-acting form when the daily insulin requirement has been assessed. The insulin requirements of such patients may increase suddenly during stress and acute illness, precipitating the onset of ketoacidosis if the insulin dosage is not matched to the patient's requirements. Many cases of diabetic coma are initiated by failure to increase insulin dosage during acute illness, and are largely avoidable. Once developed, diabetic coma requires careful and rapid treatment with short-acting insulin, and large quantities of fluid and electrolytes; the severe acidosis and the substantial deficits of sodium, potassium, and water, must be adequately corrected during the early stages of treatment.

1. Cahill, G. F., Owen, E. O., Felig, P., Morgan, A. P. *in* Progress in Endocrinology (edited by C. Gual); p. 148. Amsterdam, 1969.
2. Steiner, D. F., Clark, J. L., Nolan, C., Rubenstein, A. H., Margoliash, E., Aten, B., Oyer, P. E. *Rec. Prog. Horm. Res.* 1969, **25**, 207.
3. Roth, J., Gorden, P., Pasten, I. *Proc. natn. Acad. Sci. U.S.A.* 1968, **61**, 138.
4. Porte, D. *in* Progress in Endocrinology (edited by C. Gual); p. 192. Amsterdam, 1969.
5. Curry, D. L., Bennett, L. L., Grodsky, G. M. *Fedn Proc.* 1968, **27**, 496.
6. Malaisse, W., Malaisse-Lagai, F., Wright, P. H. *Endocrinology*, 1967, **80**, 99.
7. McIntyre, N., Holdsworth, C. W., Turner, D. S. *J. clin. Endocr. Metab.* 1965, **25**, 1317.
8. Perley, M. J., Kipnis, D. M. *J. clin. Invest.* 1967, **46**, 1954.
9. Unger, R. H., Ketterer, H., Dupré, J., Eisentraut, A. M. *ibid.* p. 630.
10. Marks, V., Samols, E *in* Recent Advances in Endocrinology (edited by V. H. T. James); p. 111. Boston, 1968.

11. Chisholm, D. J., Lazarus, L., Young, J. D., Kraegen, E. *Diabetes*, 1970, **19**, suppl. 1, p. 365.
12. Kraegen, E. W., Chisholm, D. J., Young, J. D., Lazarus, L. *J. clin. Invest.* 1970, **49**, 524.
13. Yalow, R. S., Berson, S. A. *ibid.*, 1960, **39**, 1157.
14. Zierler, K. L., Rabinowitz, D. *Medicine, Baltimore*, 1963, **42**, 385.
15. Siperstein, M. D., Unger, R. H., Madison, L. L. *in* Progress in Endocrinology (edited by C. Gual); p. 1136. Amsterdam, 1969.
16. Prout, T. E., Goldner, M. G. *Diabetes*, 1970, **19**, suppl. 1, p. 375.

CHAPTER NINE

Endocrine Changes During Pregnancy

EACH stage of the reproductive process depends upon the integrated actions of several hormonal control mechanisms. The control of the menstrual cycle has already been described, together with the endocrine mechanisms responsible for the hormonal regulation of sexual function, acting via L.H. to regulate steroid secretion by the gonads and via F.S.H. to produce maturation of ovarian follicles in the female and sperm development in the male. The gonadal steroids cause the development of secondary sexual characteristics (genital maturation, hair distribution, and body build) and are necessary for the adequate development of psychosexual attitudes and libido.

Once fertilisation has occurred in the oviduct, there is a high probability of implantation and development of the zygote in the œstrogen-progesterone-primed endometrium. At this stage the initiation and continuation of the pregnancy depend on corpus-luteum function, which must be maintained for several weeks to provide the steroid secretion necessary during early gestation. After this time, the placenta begins to elaborate large quantities of steroids and becomes the major source of hormones necessary for maintenance of the pregnancy. Hypophysectomy or oophorectomy do not usually cause abortion after the first trimester. During pregnancy, extensive effects on fetal and maternal endocrine function are caused by the massive secretion of steroid hormones from the placenta. Various œstrogen-dependent binding proteins are increased in the maternal plasma during pregnancy, and the secretion of certain pituitary hormones is inhibited. Characteristic changes occur in the renin-angiotensin system, and aldosterone secretion from the maternal adrenal is increased.

Mammary development is stimulated in preparation for lactation, and changes in carbohydrate tolerance occur in women whose insulin secretory capacity is impaired. In the fetus, characteristic metabolic transformation of œstrogens and progesterone occur, and the fetal tissues are in contact with high concentrations of steroid hormones throughout pregnancy and for the first few days of life.

Hormones and Sexual Function

Sexual behaviour patterns in animals are usually regulated by the effects of gonadal steroids secreted in response to hypothalamic-pituitary rhythms and are related to seasonal factors or characteristic ovarian cycles. In man, steroid hormones are equally necessary as a background for sexual behaviour, but they have a relatively small effect on the frequency and timing of sexual activity, except at the extremes of concentration—e.g., the decline in potency and libido which follows failure of pituitary or testicular function, and the enhanced libido which accompanies androgen excess. In the male, testosterone is necessary for the development and maintenance of libido and potency. Once developed, libido may be retained despite the development of moderate androgen deficiency, though there is usually some decline in potency when androgen secretion is impaired. The decline in sexual potency which occurs with ageing in the male is not due to androgen lack, since testosterone secretion remains fairly constant with advancing years. In men with true androgen deficiency, testosterone replacement causes dramatic improvement in libido and wellbeing; in psychogenic impotence, testosterone secretion is usually normal and androgen treatment has little effect. An important clinical distinction between the two conditions is that androgen-deficient men rarely complain of impotence, whereas patients with psychogenic impotence are deeply concerned about the symptom. There is evidence that testosterone secretion may be more immediately concerned with sexual function than was formerly appreciated; testosterone secretion has been found to rise in men during periods of increased sexual activity, and some patients with psychogenic impotence have shown reduced plasma-testosterone. Œstrogen administration in men causes a striking decline in libido and potency, owing to inhibition of pituitary L.H. secretion and reduced testosterone secretion.

In the female, gonadal steroids have less clearcut effects on sexual activity, whereas androgen secretion by the adrenal seems to be a major factor in promoting libido. Pituitary or adrenal failure is followed by loss of libido, whereas ovarian failure has relatively less effect on sexual function. Excess androgen is sometimes accompanied by enhanced libido, as in women treated with testosterone analogues, while œstrogen and progesterone have relatively little effect on the intensity of the libido. However, œstrogen secretion maintains normal genital function in the female and is to this extent an important contributing factor to sexual activity. Although high rates of œstrogen secretion are associated with œstrous behaviour and sexual receptivity in most other vertebrate species, there is little evidence for œstrogen-programmed sexual activity in the human female. Some women notice increased libido at the time of the mid-cycle preovulatory œstrogen peak, and others experience reduced sexual interest during the luteal phase when progesterone secretion is maximum. In general, psychic factors are of predominant importance in the patterns of human sexual behaviour, while the steroid hormones maintain the necessary genital development and libido which provide the background for sexual function.

In some species, clearcut hormonal events are stimulated by coitus and influence the subsequent course of pregnancy—e.g., in rodents, coitus and cervical stimulation are followed by pituitary release of prolactin, which stimulates corpus-luteum formation and progesterone secretion. There is no definite evidence for coitus-induced hormonal effects in primates, though relatively few studies have been done.

Control of Corpus-luteum Function

The earliest stages of pregnancy depend on the secretion of optimum levels of œstrogen and progesterone by the corpus luteum. For implantation to occur, migration of the blastocyst down the fallopian tube must be integrated with the development of the uterine endometrium and the activity of the myometrium. Tubal migration is influenced by œstrogens, and both œstrogens and progesterone are necessary for development of the secretory endometrium. The provision of adequate levels of each steroid at the appropriate time is necessary for successful implantation, which occurs about 7 days after ovulation, at the time of maximum œstradiol and progesterone secretion. After implantation, continued secretion of progesterone is essential for maintenance of the established pregnancy. Progesterone secretion at first originates from the corpus luteum, which has a functional life of 8 to 10 weeks during early pregnancy, in contrast to the usual life span of 2 weeks when pregnancy does not occur. Progesterone secretion shows an initial rise and a transient fall with the decline of corpus-luteum function after the first few weeks of pregnancy, then rises again as the placental secretion of progesterone becomes established.

Since implantation depends on the provision of an optimum steroid-hormone milieu by the corpus luteum, it is probable that some cases of implantation failure are due to defective corpus-luteum function. The occurrence of short luteal phases with evidence of deficient corpus-luteum function is seen in about 10% of ovulatory cycles and is believed to be a contributing factor to infertility. In such patients, the luteal phase lasts only 10 days or less, instead of the usual 13 days or more; secretion of 17OH-progesterone, progesterone, and œstrogen is reduced, and menstruation occurs as early as 6–8 days after the L.H. peak. This fault in corpus-luteum function is probably due to inadequate F.S.H. secretion during the preceding follicular phase, leading through deficient follicular development to impaired luteinisation and function of the corpus luteum.[1]

Comparative studies have shown the presence of various luteotrophic factors in different animal species—prolactin in rodents, œstrogen in rabbits, and L.H. in sheep have all been shown to maintain the corpus luteum. Also, luteolytic hormones of uterine origin have been thought cause cessation of corpus-luteum function in some species. In sheep there is evidence that prostaglandin release from the uterus may be responsible for the termination of corpus-luteum activity.

In primates, there is no clear evidence for the existence of luteotrophic or luteolytic factors, and the corpus luteum seems to have an intrinsic life span of 8 to 10 weeks in the presence of an early pregnancy. Luteotrophic factors may be produced by the blastocyst, but, in man, the factor most likely to be responsible for maintaining corpus-luteum function is human chorionic gonadotrophin (H.C.G.). This protein hormone is formed by the trophoblast as soon as implantation occurs, stimulating the development of the corpus luteum and its secretion of steroids during the first few weeks after fertilisation. However, H.C.G. does not have a continuing effect on the corpus luteum, which begins to show declining steroid secretion after some 4 weeks, despite the rising secretion of H.C.G. to peak levels several weeks later.

This evanescence of corpus-luteum function is responsible for the biphasic pattern of progesterone secretion in early pregnancy. During the normal cycle, plasma-progesterone rises from low levels in the follicular phase to a peak at the middle of the luteal phase, and declines again before menstruation. When pregnancy occurs, plasma-progesterone rises sharply to a much higher peak 3–4 weeks after ovulation, then declines to a nadir 40–50 days after ovulation, before rising again and showing a continuous increase throughout the rest of pregnancy. The initial rise and fall are due to the development and decline of corpus-luteum function, and the secondary rise reflects progesterone production by the placenta. By term, placental secretion of progesterone rises to 250 mg. per day, from basal levels of 25 mg. per day during the luteal phase of the non-pregnant female.

Whereas plasma-progesterone reflects the combined secretory activities of corpus-luteum and placenta during early pregnancy, the function of the corpus luteum alone can be assessed by measurement of plasma-17 OH-progesterone, which is not secreted by the placenta.[2] During the first 5 weeks after implantation plasma-levels of 17 OH-progesterone and progesterone rise and fall together. However, 17 OH-progesterone levels continue to fall towards basal levels when progesterone levels are again rising after the nadir at 6–7 weeks, reflecting the limited functional life of the corpus luteum and the change-over from corpus luteum to placenta as the source of progesterone during pregnancy (fig. 33).

Actions of Progesterone

Progesterone has an essential role with œstradiol in implantation and is thereafter the major hormonal factor in the maintenance of pregnancy. It causes the œstrogen-stimulated proliferative endometrium to undergo secretory changes which permit implantation of the fertilised ovum, and it suppresses myometrial activity to allow retention of the established pregnancy. In some animals, the corpus luteum continues to secrete progesterone throughout pregnancy, and oophorectomy results in abortion unless progesterone replacement is given. In human beings there is an increased risk of abortion at the time of the second missed period, corresponding to the nadir of plasma-progesterone and probably due to decline of progesterone below a critical minimum level during the transition phase between corpus luteum and placenta. However, the shift of progesterone synthesis from the corpus luteum to the placenta renders the pregnancy relatively independent of ovarian function after the first few weeks; for this reason, oophorectomy as early as the second or third month does not usually affect the course of pregnancy.

The extremely high secretion-rate of progesterone results in high concentration of the steroid in the fetal membranes and myometrium,

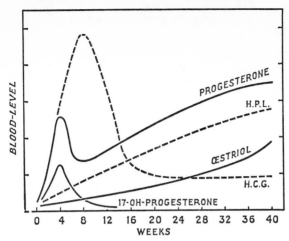

Fig. 33—Profiles of hormone production by the corpus luteum and placenta during normal pregnancy.

where it exerts a local blocking action upon myometrial activity, allowing only non-propagated asynchronous activity of the uterus, despite its considerably increased working potential.[3] Comparable effects occur during the luteal phase of the normal menstrual cycle, rendering the uterus most quiescent when the possibility of implantation is highest. The fall in progesterone secretion after mid-cycle is followed by an increase in uterine muscle activity during menstruation, consistent with the view that a fall of progesterone level leads to enhanced myometrial contractility. If fertilisation occurs, plasma-progesterone continues to rise after the mid-cycle, and uterine activity reaches a minimum during the earliest stages of implantation and placental development. The declining plasma-progesterone level at term has been thought to trigger the onset of labour; this mechanism seems to operate in the rabbit, but is less clearcut in man. Progesterone withdrawal is not thought to be the main factor in the onset of labour in primates, and it is likely that the effects of plasma-progesterone level and uterine volume contribute in different degrees to the initiation of labour in different species. In rabbits, the progesterone factor is dominant, whereas in man it may operate in conjunction with the rate of change in intrauterine volume and is much less clearly correlated with the onset of labour. The human placenta seems to have an intrinsic life span and to become increasingly sensitive to oxytocin, volume change, and progesterone level as term approaches. After delivery of the placenta, the maternal progesterone levels quickly fall back to those of the non-pregnant state.

Progesterone is converted by the maternal tissues to various metabolites which are excreted principally in the urine, mainly as conjugates to glucuronic acid. The excretion of pregnanediol glucuronide in urine has been widely used as an index of progesterone secretion during clinical studies, though it is not derived solely from the metabolism of progesterone. More accurate measures of progesterone production rates have been obtained by the use of metabolic clearance-rate determinations but are not necessary for clinical evaluation and management. Plasma-progesterone levels during pregnancy can now be rapidly measured by a simple binding assay and provide an excellent index of progesterone secretion by the corpus luteum and placenta.[4]

Protein Hormones of the Placenta

The placenta secretes two protein hormones in high concentrations into the maternal circulation. H.C.G. is a glycoprotein (M.W. 30,000) with a high content of sialic acid and other carbohydrate residues which seem to be essential for the biological activity of the protein. The trophoblast begins to secrete H.C.G. as soon as implantation occurs; the hormone can be detected in plasma and urine by radioimmunoassay as early as 9 days after fertilisation and is present in the fetus as well as in the maternal circulation. H.C.G. is actively concentrated by the cells of the corpus luteum, causing it to persist and secrete increasing quantities of steroids during the first few weeks of pregnancy. Secretion of H.C.G. rises to a peak at 60–80 days, then declines as the cytotrophoblast cells of the placenta become less numerous (fig. 33). Although the initial persistence and steroid secretion of the corpus luteum are due to H.C.G., the corpus luteum reaches a peak of hormone secretion 3–4 weeks after fertilisation and then becomes progressively less active, despite the rising levels of H.C.G., until 9–12 weeks. The role of H.C.G. in pregnancy seems to be confined to its transient stimulating effect on the corpus luteum. The similar effects of H.C.G. and L.H. on the stimulation of steroidogenesis are related to structural similarities between the two hormones. Both proteins consist of two subunits, which display substantial homology of sequence between the two hormones, and also to some extent with the subunits of T.S.H. and F.S.H. H.C.G. has been widely used as a substitute for human pituitary L.H. in clinical conditions requiring gonadal stimulation, in particular for stimulation of testis function and for triggering ovulation (from follicles previously developed by F.S.H. administration) in the treatment of infertility. The other major protein hormone of the placenta is human placental lactogen (H.P.L.) or chorionic somatomammotrophin (H.C.S.), which is secreted in increasing quantities by the syncytiotrophoblast cells from the first few weeks of pregnancy until term. H.C.S. has no resemblance to H.C.G.; it contains no carbohydrate residues, being a simple protein chain (M.W. 18,500) with notable structural similarities to H.G.H. H.C.S. does not possess significant biological growth activity but cross-reacts with antibodies to human growth hormone. It has striking prolactin-like activity in various animal systems and causes impaired carbohydrate tolerance in animals with reduced insulin secretory capacity. Secretion of H.C.S. rises substantially as pregnancy proceeds, reaching blood-levels of several microgrammes per ml. at term, with a secretion-rate of over 1 g. daily. The exact function of H.C.S. is not known, but it has been thought to promote energy supply to the fetus by providing free fatty acids for maternal metabolism and sparing glucose and protein for utilisation by the fetus.[5] The secretion-rate of H.C.S. provides an index of placental function and may be useful in the management of toxæmic and other pregnancies in which there is an increased risk to the fetus. There is a correlation between placental mass and the H.C.S. level in plasma, and placental size seems largely to determine the amount of H.C.S. produced during pregnancy. There is very little transfer of H.C.S. into the fetal circulation, where its concentration is only 1% of the level in maternal blood. Although H.C.S. has relatively small intrinsic growth-hormone-like activity, the very high levels which occur in blood during late pregnancy may act indirectly as a growth hormone for the fetus by sparing glucose utilisation in the mother. Since the fetus is extremely dependent on glucose for metabolism, H.C.S.-induced insulin resistance and mobilisation of free fatty acids for maternal utilisation would provide glucose to the fetus during the period of maximum growth in late pregnancy.

Biosynthesis and Metabolism of Steroid Hormones in the Fetoplacental Unit

There are considerable differences in the steroid-secretion patterns of different species during pregnancy, and the human fetoplacental unit displays unique features of steroid metabolism and interconversion (fig. 34). The fetus and placenta both possess incomplete pathways for steroid biosynthesis and are complementary to each other in the synthesis and metabolism of progesterone, œstrogen, androgen, and corticosteroids.[6] The human placenta synthesises massive quantities of progesterone from maternal cholesterol, transferring up to 75 mg. progesterone daily to the fetus, while the remainder is metabolised by maternal tissues. The placenta also supplies pregnenolone to the fetus, and transfers steroids such as D.H.A. from the maternal adrenal. Large quantities of progesterone are metabolised by the fetal tissues, either to inactive derivatives or to the steroids produced by the adrenals and testis. Pregnenolone is converted by the fetal adrenal to Δ^5 androgens which pass back to the placenta and comprise the major precursor for œstrogen formation during pregnancy.

The placenta has important functional relations with the fetal adrenals, which are notable for the presence of a pituitary-dependent hypertrophic inner cell layer (the "fetal zone") and for the absence of the enzymes necessary for conversion of Δ^5 to Δ^4 steroids. The fetal adrenal is therefore unable to convert Δ^5 precursors such as pregnenolone into progesterone and its derivatives and is dependent on the placenta for progesterone for the synthesis of adrenal steroids. Large quantities of Δ^5 pregnenolone are converted in the fetal adrenal to androgen precursors such as dehydroepiandrosterone (D.H.A.) sulphate, some of which is hydroxylated in the fetal liver to form 16 hydroxy D.H.A. sulphate.[7]

In the placenta, the Δ^5 sulphates are hydrolysed, converted to Δ^4 androgens, and rapidly aromatised to form œstradiol and œstriol The large amounts of œstradiol formed from D.H.A. by the placenta are metabolised extensively by the fetus, mainly by 16 hydroxylation to œstriol and by a 15 hydroxylation pathway which is unique to the fetus. Most of the œstriol excreted by the mother is formed from 16 OH-D.H.A. originating in the fetal adrenal cortex and from the metabolism of œstradiol by fetal tissues. Œstriol levels in maternal plasma and urine are therefore a valuable index of fetal metabolism and viability, and are greatly reduced by fetal death in utero. Œstriol levels are also very low in pregnancies with anencephalic fetuses, which often have hypoplastic adrenal glands.

The progesterone secreted by the placenta into the fetal circulation is largely metabolised by the adrenals, liver, and other tissues. In the adrenal, it is converted into various hydroxylated steroids, especially

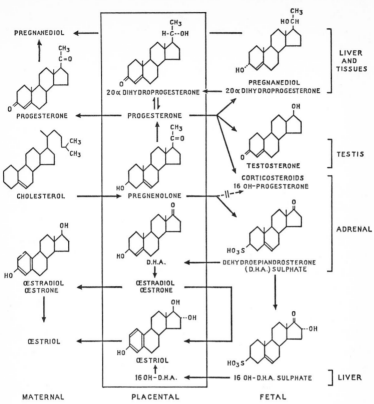

Fig. 34—Steroid-hormone metabolism by the maternal, placental, and fetal tissues at mid-pregnancy.

16 OH-progesterone. It can also be utilised by the fetal adrenal gland for corticosteroid synthesis, and by the fetal testis for testosterone synthesis; the fetal ovary is relatively inactive in steroidogenesis and converts progesterone only to 20α-dihydroprogesterone.

In the fetal liver, progesterone is actively metabolised to 20α-dihydroprogesterone and pregnanediol and conjugated to form sulphates and glucuronides. Other fetal tissues also metabolise progesterone actively, forming 20α-dihydroprogesterone and other derivatives. The large quantities of 20α-dihydroprogesterone formed in the fetus are reconverted to progesterone in the placenta, providing a mechanism whereby the steroid is recovered after passage through the fetus. This process presumably allows high progesterone levels in the maternal tissues, with lower levels of the active steroid in the fetus. The large quantities of œstrogen formed in the placenta are also substantially metabolised by the fetus, by hydroxylation to inactive deriatives and sulphation to enhance water solubility and excretion.

The Fetal Endocrine System

The development of certain of the fetal endocrine organs has been briefly described in previous chapters. All endocrine glands are well developed by the end of the first trimester, and the secretion of A.C.T.H. and growth hormone from the fetal pituitary has already begun at this time. During embryonic life, the fetal adrenal and gonads secrete steroid hormones and precursors, as already described. The development of the gonad into functional testis or ovary is determined by the sex chromosomes of the fetus, whereas the development of the genitalia depends on the presence or absence of androgen and an additional testicular inhibitor of the müllerian-duct system. The fetal gonads are formed when the mesodermal gonadal ridges containing the primitive sex cords are invaded by the primordial germ-cells. The gonad is at first similar in the male and female, and the germ-cells probably have the potential to form either sperm or ova. Between 6 and 8 weeks the gonad differentiates into a testis or ovary and determines the subsequent development of the genital tract from the coexisting wolffian and müllerian duct systems.

In male embryos the medullary portion of the indifferent gonad proliferates, and the sex cords develop into the immature seminiferous tubules. Leydig cells develop from the interstitial mesenchymal cells of the early testis and become functional by the 8th week of development. Although the germ-cell component of the testis remains quiescent until puberty, the interstitial cells are active during early fetal life, reaching a peak of androgen production during the 4th month. This activity may be caused by the action of H.C.G. on the fetal testis but seems to be at least partly dependent on pituitary control.

Early steroidogenesis is a feature of the fetal testis in many species and seems to be an important stimulus to the development of the wolffian-duct systems into the male genitalia. The fetal testis is also responsible for suppression of the müllerian-duct systems; testosterone is not involved in this inhibition, which is caused by an organiser or inducer produced by the testis and acting locally to suppress the adjacent müllerian duct.

The developmental features of the fetal ovary are almost the opposite of those of the testis and occur several weeks later. The ovary develops from the cortical portion of the indifferent gonad, and is extremely active in germ-cell multiplication, with little steroidogenesis. The full complement of female gametes is present in the gonad during fetal life, whereas those of the male do not develop until puberty. The development of the female genital system does not depend on the presence of the gonad, for the müllerian ducts differentiate spontaneously into the internal genitalia, and the wolffian system regresses in the absence of androgen.

The external genitalia develop from a common structural anlage with the potential for differentiation into either male or female genitals. Here again, the influence of androgen is paramount in determining the direction and extent of differentiation from the innate female pattern to that of the male. Androgen deprivation will cause the male fetus to develop female external as well as internal genitalia; removal of the ovary does not influence the differentiation of the female genitalia, whereas androgen administration causes varying degrees of masculinisation of the genitalia of the female fetus.

Maternal Changes During Pregnancy

The high output of steroid and protein hormones from the placenta produces a variety of maternal changes during pregnancy. Most of these effects are due to high levels of plasma-œstrogen, which stimulates the synthesis of several proteins by the liver. Among these are a group of hormone-transport proteins: sex-hormone-binding globulin (S.H.B.G. or TE B.G.), which binds œstrogens and androgens, is sharply increased and probably helps to minimise the level of free œstrogen in the circulation. Cortisol-binding globulin (C.B.G.) and thyroxine-binding globulin (T.B.G.) are also increased, resulting in high plasma-levels of cortisol and thyroxine. Because of the enhanced binding of these hormones, their physiologically effective free levels are not greatly increased, and features of hormone excess do not develop.

The formation of renin substrate by the liver is also increased by œstrogens, resulting in an elevation of plasma-renin activity during pregnancy and a rise in the plasma-antigiotensin-II level. There is an accompanying rise in aldosterone secretion and excretion as pregnancy progresses; although this rise in aldosterone secretion may be due partly to the elevation of plasma-angiotensin, it may also be related to the inhibitory effect of high concentrations of progesterone and its hydroxylated derivatives on sodium retention by the renal tubule. High concentrations of renin are present in the pregnant uterus and the amniotic fluid but do not contribute to the maternal plasma-renin level and do not have a demonstrable local action upon the uterus and its contents.

Endocrine Factors in Parturition

There does not seem to be a clearcut endocrine mechanism which controls the onset of labour. The roles of progesterone withdrawal and increasing uterine volume have been outlined above; neither seems adequate to explain the initiation of labour, which operates as though related to an intrinsic life span of the placenta. Oxytocin is probably important in enhancing uterine contractions once parturition has begun, but it is not necessary for the onset of labour. Delivery can be successful in patients and animals with deficient neurohypophyseal function and total absence of oxytocin. On the other hand, the myometrium becomes increasingly sensitive to oxytocin as term approaches, and oxytocin release may sometimes cause premature contractions. It is secreted in the later stages of normal labour and may facilitate delivery and contraction of the uterus.[1]

Other endocrine factors have been implicated in the initiation of labour, including corticosteroid levels and the local formation of angiotensin by the action of uterine renin. There is no convincing evidence for either of these proposals, and the levels of angiotensin II in amniotic fluid remain unchanged during the onset of labour. Plasma-levels of prostaglandins rise during labour but have not been proved to be causally related to the initiation of labour.

Lactation

In women, mammary development requires the direct actions of œstrogen, progesterone, and pituitary hormones, and the presence of basal levels of thyroxine, cortisol, and insulin. Œstrogen causes development of the mammary ducts, and progesterone stimulates formation of lobules and alveoli. Optimum mammary growth in animals also requires the presence of growth hormone and prolactin. In women, normal breast development is initiated by œstrogen, progesterone, and growth hormone. During pregnancy, the high levels of œstrogen and progesterone induce alveolar development, in synergy with the stimulating effect of H.C.S. Although H.C.S. is lactogenic in other species, it does not cause milk secretion in the human female during pregnancy.

In other species, prolactin is a well-defined protein of the anterior pituitary, and is normally kept under inhibitory control by the hypothalamus. Prolactin levels are higher in females than in males and are stimulated by œstrogen; after delivery, prolactin levels rise considerably and initiate lactation. In man, such clearcut evidence about prolactin has only recently been found. Prolactin has never been satisfactorily isolated from the human pituitary, except in the form of prolactin-rich growth-hormone preparations. However, various pieces of evidence indicate that prolactin is secreted by the human pituitary under appropriate conditions. Bioassay studies have shown the presence of prolactin activity in urine during lactation, and a sensitive plasma bioassay has detected prolactin in the blood of lactating women, patients with acromegaly and inappropriate lactation, and patients on phenothiazine therapy (which stimulates prolactin release from the pituitary). Recent radioimmunoassay studies have shown that plasma-prolactin rises progressively during pregnancy, falls after delivery, and rises again during breast-feeding. During pregnancy and lactation specific acidophil cells with characteristic staining and large granules are demonstrable in the human pituitary. These cells are not present at other times and have been proposed as the prolactin-secreting cells of the hypophysis. Their appearance is accompanied by a reduction in the number of somatotrophs in the pituitary, consistent with the impairment of maternal growth-hormone secretion during pregnancy. The massive secretion of H.C.S. and œstrogens from the placenta probably leads to suppression of G.H. secretion by the pituitary. The high œstrogen level may also stimulate the development of the prolactin-secreting cells as in other species, possibly from a common precursor cell of the acidophil series.

1. Ross, G. T. *Rec. Prog. Horm. Res.* 1970, **26**, 1.
2. Lipsett, M. B., Cargille, C. M., Ross, G. T. *Ann. intern. Med.* 1970, **72**, 933.
3. Csapo, A. I., Wood, C. *in* Recent Advances in Endocrinology (edited by V. H. T. James); p. 207. Boston, 1968.

4. Johansson, E. D. B. *in* Karolinska Symposium on Methods in Reproductive Biology (edited by E. Diczfalusy); p. 188. Stockholm, 1970.
5. Grumbach, M. M., Kaplan, S. L., Sciarra, J. J., Burr, J. M. *Ann. N. Y. Acad. Sci.* 1968, **148**, 591.
6. Villee, D. B. *New Engl. J. Med.* 1969, **281**, 473.
7. Solomon, S., Bird, C. E., Ling, W., Iwamija, M., Young, P. C. M. *Rec. Prog. Horm. Res.* 1967, **23**, 297.

CHAPTER TEN

Endocrine-Function Tests

THE functional states of endocrine glands are most accurately evaluated by measurement of the rates at which they produce hormones. In addition to measurement of the basal level of hormone secretion, the response to stimulation and suppression gives valuable information about the secretory capacity of the gland and its responsiveness to normal regulatory mechanisms. Although this theoretical ideal can now be reached for most endocrine glands, the exact measurement of hormone-secretion rate is usually a complex procedure, involving administration of radioactive isotopes to the patient and careful collection of blood and urine samples for analysis. Secretion-rate measurements are more often used for investigation of hormonal physiology and metabolism than for diagnosis. Endocrine function is most commonly evaluated by procedures which measure aspects of the metabolism or action of the hormone being studied. Endocrine-function tests formerly relied on assay of hormones and their metabolites in urine, by bioassay or chemical assay. More sensitive assays and improved specificity led to the measurement of hormones in blood, which remains the most useful approach to endocrine diagnosis and management.

Indirect tests of hormone activity were used for clinical assessment of endocrine disorders before the advent of specific methods of hormone measurement; alterations in the metabolism of sugar, lipid, salt, and water provide useful supplementary data about hormonal disturbances but are neither specific nor sensitive indices of endocrine function. In some instances, as in the thyroidal uptake and turnover of iodine-131, radioactive precursors can be used to study the activity of endocrine glands.

Most methods of estimating endocrine function rely on the measurement of blood or urine levels of hormones. Secretion-rate measurement is largely performed as a research procedure, and the indirect tests of hormone activity are used mainly to supplement more specific methods of hormone assay.

Methods of Hormone Assay

The methodology of hormone assay has changed greatly in the past 15 years, with the introduction of more sensitive and specific procedures. Chemical and physical assay methods were applicable to compounds of characteristic physicochemical properties and adequate concentration in blood or urine. Thus, plasma-protein-bound-iodine (P.B.I.) gives a measure of the circulating thyroid-hormone level, and urinary corticosteroids and ketosteroids reflect adrenal hormone secretion. Among the indirect tests, serum-calcium provides a valuable indirect measure of parathyroid function, and blood-sugar levels are useful indicators of pancreatic endocrine function.

The earliest hormone assays were bioassays, based on the specific response of hormone-sensitive tissues in a test animal. For hormones of well-defined and relatively simple structure, physical and chemical methods of measurement were developed to replace bioassay. In chemical reactions involving radioactive reagents, the labelled derivatives can be isolated and counted, providing a highly sensitive method of assay. Another advantage of isotopic assay methods is that a labelled form of the hormone can be used to correct losses during the extraction and assay procedure.

The most important group of assay procedures now in use involve the displacement of labelled hormone from a specific binding protein by unlabelled hormone. Increasing amounts of unlabelled hormone cause proportionate decreases in attachment of the radioactive hormone to the specific binding protein, and can be estimated by reference to a standard curve. The procedure is called "radioimmunoassay" when specific antibody is used as the binding protein,[1] and "protein-binding assay" when naturally occurring transport or receptor proteins are used.[2] The two versions are essentially similar and have also been called "saturation analysis".[3]

Assay Procedures

Bioassay

Biological assays have been of great value in the purification and isolation of protein hormones. Classical bioassays are not generally sensitive enough to measure hormones in body-fluids, but more sensitive versions are being developed.

Growth hormone.—Administration of G.H. to hypophysectomised rats causes body growth and widening of the tibial epiphysis in proportion to the dose administered. This assay is not sensitive enough for measurement of G.H. in body-fluids but is the standard assay for pituitary-G.H. preparations used in clinical treatment and research.

Prolactin.—The hypertrophic response of the pigeon crop sac and lactogenic activity in rabbits have been used for assay. The lactogenic response of mouse mammary glands in organ culture has been developed into a sensitive assay for blood-prolactin activity.

Gonadotrophins.—F.S.H. is asayed by its stimulating action on ovarian weight in H.C.G.-treated rats; L.H. and H.C.G. are also assayed in the rat, by their effects on depletion of ovarian ascorbic acid in the female or growth of the prostate in the male, both effects being manifestations of increased steroid secretion by the gonads. For clinical use, the uterine-growth response of the immature mouse provides a useful index of the total gonadotrophin content of urine. Low levels occur in hypopituitarism and in selective impairment of gonadotrophin secretion, and high values are found in primary gonadal failure.

A.C.T.H.—Adrenal ascorbic-acid depletion and corticosteroid secretion have been used for bioassay of A.C.T.H. preparations. These methods have also been used to establish blood-A.C.T.H. levels in pituitary-adrenal disorders (levels are low in hypopituitarism and high in Addison's disease). Though used intensively by a few laboratories, the methods for blood-A.C.T.H. bioassay are too demanding for general use. A much more sensitive bioassay, using the steroidogenic response of isolated adrenal cells, has lately been developed.

Thyrotrophin.—The most sensitive bioassay depends on the release of labelled thyroid hormone from the thyroid of mice previously treated with radio-iodine. This assay detects T.S.H. in plasma and also the long-acting thyroid stimulator (L.A.T.S.) which is associated with thyrotoxicosis.

Insulin.—Bioassays for insulin include those based on its hypoglycæmic effect in mice, its effect on glucose uptake by the rat diaphragm in vitro, and the acceleration of rat-adipose-tissue metabolism in vitro.

Glucagon.—Activation of adenyl cyclase in liver extracts.

Vasopressin.—Antidiuretic effect in alcohol-treated rats.

Oxytocin.—Contraction of rat uterus.

Angiotensin.—Blood-pressure response of the ganglion-blocked rat, or contraction of the superfused rat colon.

Chemical and Physical Assay

The formation of chemical derivatives with characteristic chromogenic or fluorescent properties can be used for chemically unique hormones of sufficient concentration in body-fluids—e.g., steroids, and thyroxine as measured by protein-bound iodine.

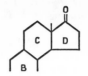

Fig. 35—Reactive group for the   ig. 36—Reactive group for
Porter-Silber reaction.   the Zimmerman reaction.

Porter-Silber reaction for 17-hydroxycorticosteroids.—Phenylhydrazine forms a characteristic brown chromogen with steroids carrying the dihydroxyacetone group on ring D. This reaction measures cortisol, cortisone, and most of their metabolites and is used for measuring adrenal steroids in urine and blood (fig. 35).

Zimmerman reaction for 17-ketosteroids.—Metadinitrobenzene forms a purple chromogen with steroids carrying a ketone group in the 17 position (fig. 36). This method measures a variety of ketosteroids derived from the adrenal and testis and is only occasionally of diagnostic value in its original form. However, the Zimmerman reaction can also be used to measure urinary corticosteroids after conversion of cortisol metabolites to 17-ketosteroids by oxidation of the side chain. The ketogenic steroids estimated in this way include a variety of steroid metabolites, and can account for the majority of the cortisol normally secreted by the adrenal, as well as pregnanetriol excreted by patients with congenital adrenal hyperplasia.

Fluorimetric assay of steroids can be done in acid or alkaline solutions. The acid fluorescence test has been developed into a useful assay for the rapid measurement of plasma-cortisol in clinical practice .[4]

Mass detection.—Measurement by the mass-detection device of the gas-liquid chromatography apparatus has been used to assay the blood-levels of some steroids, particularly pregnanediol and testosterone.

Isotope Derivative Assay

Reaction of steroids with radioactive compounds such as ^{3}H-acetic anhydride of known specific activity (d.p.m. per μmole) leads to the formation of labelled steroid acetates which can be isolated by paper chromatography and counted to determine the mass of steroid (fig. 37). Losses of steroids during the extraction and isolation procedures can be corrected by observing the recovery of ^{14}C-labelled steroid added to the original blood-sample.[5] This method has been particularly applied to the estimation of cortisol, corticosterone, aldosterone, and testosterone in blood and urine.

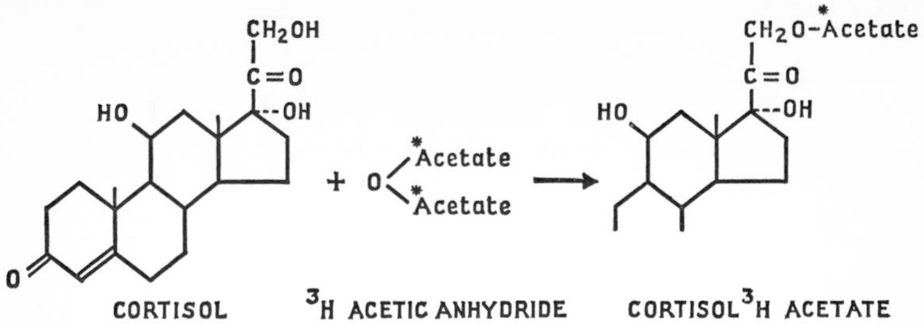

Fig. 37—*Formation of labelled steroid derivative by acetylation with tritiated acetic anhydride.*

If the acetic anhydride specific activity (d.p.m. per μmole) is known, the radio-activity (d.p.m.) of cortisol acetate isolated by chromatography can be used to calculate the mass of steroid (μmole) isolated. Purification losses can be completely corrected by determining the recovery of ^{14}C-cortisol added to each plasma sample.

Saturation Analysis

This term refers to a rapidly expanding group of techniques which use the ability of certain binding proteins to combine specifically with a usually smaller molecule, the ligand. Examples of such binding pairs are: all antigen-antibody reactions, the binding of thyroxine, cortisol, and gonadal hormones to specific plasma-globulins, and the binding of steroid and peptide hormones to their cellular receptor sites—e.g., of œstradiol to protein extracted from the uterus.

By using a labelled ligand, it is possible to set up an assay system in which the combination of binding protein and labelled ligand can be inhibited by the introduction of extremely small quantities of the unlabelled ligand. The resulting fall in protein-bound radioactivity can be used to establish a standard curve for the estimation of unknown amounts of ligand over the picogramme to nanogramme range of concentration.

Binding protein (B) + Labelled ligand (*L)
$$\rightleftharpoons \text{Protein-ligand complex (B*L)}$$
If only *L is present, then, for example: $6B + 12*L \rightleftharpoons 6B\ *L + 6*L$
If unlabelled ligand (L) is added to the system:
$$6B + 12*L + 12L \rightleftharpoons 3B*L + 3B\ L + 9*L + 9L$$
(i.e., protein-bound *L is reduced by about 50%, and the free *L is increased by 50%).

Isolation and counting of the protein-bound radioactivity, which is inversely proportional to the total mass of ligand present, gives standard curves of the form shown in fig. 38.

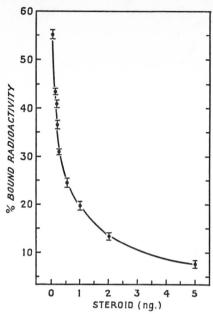

Fig. 38—Standard curve of a typical protein-binding assay.
Progressive fall in bound radioactivity occurs in the presence of increasing amounts of steroid. Similar standard curves are obtained for radioimmunoassays, which are commonly plotted as bound/free radioactivity as well as the bound/total radioactivity shown in this sample.

TABLE IV—HORMONES MEASURED BY RADIOLIGAND PROTEIN-BINDING ASSAY[2]

Source of binding protein	Hormone
Plasma-proteins	
Corticosteroid-binding globulin (C.B.G.)	Cortisol, progesterone, corticosterone, 11-desoxycortisol, 17α-hydroxyprogesterone.
Thyroxine-binding globulin (T.B.G.)	Thyroxine, triiodothyronine.
Sex-hormone-binding globulin (S.H.B.G.) or (TE B.G.)	Testosterone, œstradiol.
Cellular Receptors	
Uterine	Œstradiol, œstrone
Adrenal	A.C.T.H.
Gonadal	L.H., H.C.G.

These general properties of the saturation-analysis system have been used to establish competitive-binding assays to measure plasma-levels of hormones such as cortisol, progesterone, œstradiol, testosterone, thyroxine, and triiodothyronine (table IV). For the assay of plasma-steroids, tritiated steroids of high specific activity are used for tracer; for T3 and T4 binding assays ^{125}I-labelled thyroid hormones are used.

Radioimmunoassay

While the term "competitive-binding assay" has become accepted to describe the version of saturation analysis which uses specific binding proteins of plasma or tissue origin, the term "radioimmunoassay" has been used to describe the method in which specific antibody is used as the basis for saturation analysis. The procedure of radioimmunoassay was devised by Berson and Yalow[7] for the measurement of plasma-insulin, based on their observations on the reaction of labelled and unlabelled insulin with antibody present in the plasma of insulin-treated diabetic patients. This technique provided the first reliable method for the measurement of peptide and protein hormones in blood and has become the most extensively used procedure for hormone assay in blood. The wide application of radioimmunoassay was greatly facilitated by the development of a simple procedure by Greenwood et al.[7] for labelling peptide and protein hormones with iodine-131 and iodine-125 to high specific activity.

Although bioassay procedures have been valuable for the measurement of hormones in tissue extracts and during purification procedures, their main application to clinical studies has been in the bioassay of urinary gonadotrophin content.[8] The ascorbic-acid-depletion bioassay for blood-A.C.T.H. levels has also provided valuable information about A.C.T.H. secretion in man,[9] but in general there have been few satisfactory bioassays of plasma-peptide-hormone levels because these levels are extremely low, being in picogramme or nanogramme amounts per ml. Since the peptide hormones do not have unique chemical reactive groups, no chemical or isotopic-derivative procedure could be applied. Because antibodies to peptide hormones are usually highly specific, they can be made to react selectively with radioiodinated hormones, which are displaced by unlabelled hormone. In this way, standard curves relating the antibody-bound radioactivity to the mass of added peptide hormone can be established and used for estimation of hormone content in plasma samples. Most hormones have been found to induce satisfactory antibody formation in rabbits and guineapigs by administration in Freund's adjuvant. In some cases, coupling to carrier proteins has been used to enhance the antigenicity of hormones of low molecular weight; this procedure derives from Landsteiner's observations on hapten-induced antibody formation and has been very useful for the development of specific antibodies against relatively small molecules, such as steroids, nucleotides, and short peptides.

The original procedure of Berson and Yalow used chromatoelectrophoresis on paper strips for separation of antibody-bound and free tracer hormone. The separation of bound and free tracer has been simplified by precipitation with a second antibody to isolate the bound tracer, and adsorption to charcoal or talc to isolate free tracer. In solid-phase radioimmunoassay,[7] which simplifies isolation of the bound tracer, insoluble antibody is coupled or adsorbed to polymer in the form of particles, discs, or tubes, which are then used for radioimmunoassay. During incubation the labelled tracer becomes attached to the antibody and thus to the solid phase, which is then washed and counted to determine the bound radioactivity. Competition between the labelled and unlabelled hormone leads to a fall in the radioactivity bound to the solid phase (fig. 39). In the simplest form of this assay, sample and tracer are incubated in plastic tubes coated with antibody, which are then washed and counted to give the bound count from which the standard curve is constructed.

Linearisation of radioimmunoassay standard curves can be made by various mathematical conversions of the raw data. The easiest way is to take a reciprocal function of the bound count; this procedure is useful when the antibody is fully saturated with antigen, though logarithmic methods of transformation are more generally applicable. Both semilogarithmic and logit plots have the advantage that the slopes of standard and samples in the assay can be compared to ensure immunological identity; logit transformations are particularly useful for linearisation over the whole range of the assay.[11]

Radioimmunoassay has been applied to the measurement of many peptide and protein hormones including growth hormone. A.C.T.H., pituitary gonadotrophins, chorionic gonadotrophin, placental lactogen, insulin, glucagon, parathormone, calcitonin, gastrin, secretin, and angiotensin; the method is being increasingly used for

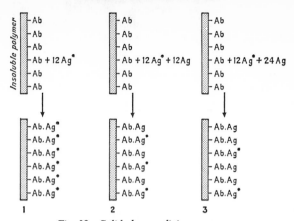

Fig. 39—Solid-phase radioimmunoassay.
(1) The antibody (Ab) attached to an insoluble polymer reacts with labelled antigen (Ag*). In the presence of increasing amounts (2) and (3) of unlabelled antigen (Ag), the radioactivity of the solid-phase complex falls in proportion to the quantity of antigen added.

the measurement of a variety of other proteins, such as immunoglobulins, and for the measurement of non-peptide hormones including œstradiol, progesterone, testosterone, aldosterone, and thyroxine. Cyclic A.M.P. has also been measured by radioimmunoassay; measurement of this nucleotide at levels encountered within the cell is of considerable importance, since cyclic A.M.P. has been implicated in the action of many hormones.

Another version of immunoassay has used labelled specific antibody for the quantitation of hormonal antigens such as insulin, G.H., and L.H. In this procedure, immunoradiometric assay, the direct reaction of antigen and antibody gives a linear increase in radioactivity with antigen mass, instead of the reciprocal fall which occurs in the conventional ligand-displacement form of immunoassay. The technique has considerable potential for the measurement of very low levels of hormones in plasma.[12]

Determination of Hormone Secretion-rates

Two approaches have been used to measure the secretion or production rate of hormones, to improve upon the unreliable estimates obtained by simple measurement of the urinary excretion of hormone metabolites. The first of these depends on the isolation of a known urinary metabolite after administration of labelled hormone, and determination of its specific activity.[13] If certain conditions are met, this value, together with the known amount of radioactivity injected, can be used to calculate the mass of endogenous hormone secreted during the period of urine collection, which should be long enough to allow complete excretion of the labelled metabolite. To estimate the secretion-rate of cortisol, a tracer dose of labelled cortisol is given, urine is collected for 48 hours, and the specific activity of tetrahydrocortisol is determined. The cortisol-secretion rate is then calculated by determining the extent of dilution of the administered labelled cortisol.

$$\frac{\text{Cortisol secretion}}{\text{during 48 hr. (}\mu\text{mole)}} = \frac{\text{Dose administered (d.p.m.)}}{\text{Specific activity of metabolite (d.p.m. per }\mu\text{mole)}}$$

In this method, the use of the cumulative activity excreted in urine integrates the plasma profile of hormone secretion throughout the period of observation.

The alternative methods are based on the concept of metabolic clearance-rate (M.C.R.), the rate at which hormone is removed from the circulation.[14] This can be measured by injection of labelled hormone followed by serial determinations of the radioactive-hormone level in plasma. The rate of disappearance of labelled hormone can be used to calculate various parameters, such as the half-life and turnover-rate, but most importantly the metabolic clearance-rate. This is calculated by dividing the administered dose of hormone by the integrated plasma radioactivity, and is measured in litres per day.

Integration of the declining radioactivity level requires multiple sampling and careful calculation. An alternative method for measuring M.C.R. uses continuous infusion of labelled hormone to achieve a constant blood-level of radioactivity. This gives a simpler and more accurate estimate of M.C.R., which is calculated by dividing the rate of infusion of labelled hormone by the stable level of hormonal radioactivity in plasma.

The M.C.R. derived by either of these methods can then be used to calculate the secretion-rate if the peripheral level of hormone is known.

Secretion-rate (μg. per day) $=$ M.C.R. (litres per day) $\times$ Peripheral level (μg. per litre)

The latter methods are most useful for the determination of production-rates during relatively short periods and have the drawback that the plasma-level of hormone must be known, and relatively constant, during the period of study. For clinical estimation of hormone-production rates, the urinary-metabolite procedure is simplest, whereas for more comprehensive studies on the production and metabolism of a hormone, the M.C.R. is very valuable. The two procedures can be combined by using constant infusion to determine M.C.R. and subsequent collection of urine for an adequate period to determine production-rate. The terms "secretion-rate" and "production-rate" are often used interchangeably, but production-rate in fact refers to the more general situation where a hormone may be formed by peripheral conversion from a precursor, as well as secreted by the gland under study. This occurs with testosterone, which in females is formed mainly by peripheral conversion from androstenedione; likewise œstradiol formation in males is largely by peripheral metabolism of androgenic precursors.

1. Yalow, R. S., Berson, S. A. *in* Protein and Polypeptide Hormones (edited by M. Margoulies); p. 36. Liége, 1968.
2. Murphy, B. E. P. *Rec. Prog. Horm. Res.* 1969, **25**, 563.
3. Ekins, R. In Vitro Procedures with Radioisotopes in Medicine; p. 325. Vienna, 1970.
4. Mattingly, D. *J. clin. Path.* 1962, **15**, 374.
5. Kliman, B., Peterson, R. E. *J. biol. Chem.* 1960, **235**, 1639.
6. Yalow, R. S., Berson S. A. *J. clin. Invest.* 1960, **39**, 1157.
7. Greenwood, F. C., Hunter, W. M., Glover, J. S. *Biochem. J.* 1963, **89**, 114.
8. Loraine, J. A., Bell, E. T. Hormone Assays and Their Clinical Application. Edinburgh, 1966.
9. Sayers, G. *in* Hormones in Blood (edited by C. H. Gray and A. L. Bacharach); p. 170. London, 1967.
10. Catt, K. J. *Acta endocr., Copenh.* 1969, **63**, suppl. 142, p. 222.
11. Rodbard, D. *ibid.* 1970, suppl. 147.
12. Miles, L. E. M., Hales, C. N. In Vitro Procedures with Radioisotopes in Medicine; p. 483. Vienna, 1970.
13. Peterson, R. E. *Rec. Prog. Horm. Res.* 1959, **15**, 231.
14. Tait, J. F., Burstein, S. *in* The Hormones (edited by G. Pincus, K. V. Thimann, and E. B. Astwood); vol. v, p. 441. New York, 1964.

Glossary

A.C.T.H.	Adrenocorticotrophic hormone, corticotrophin.
A.D.H.	Antidiuretic hormone.
A.M.P.	Adenosine monophosphate.
A.T.P.	Adenosine triphosphate.
C.B.G.	Corticosteroid-binding globulin.
C.R.F.	Corticotrophin-releasing factor
D.H.A.	Dehydroepiandrosterone.
D.I.T.	Diiodotyrosine.
D.N.A.	Deoxyribonucleic acid.
D.O.C.	Desoxycorticosterone.
F.F.A.	Free fatty acid.
F.S.H.	Follicle-stimulating hormone.
F.S.H.R.F.	Follicle-stimulating-hormone releasing factor
G.H.	Growth hormone.
G.H.R.F.	Growth-hormone releasing factor.
H.C.G.	Human chorionic gonadotrophin.
H.C.S.	Human chorionic somatomammotrophin.
H.G.H.	Human growth hormone.
H.M.G.	Human menopausal gonadotrophin.
H.P.G.	Human pituitary gonadotrophin.
H.P.L.	Human placental lactogen.
I.F.	Inhibiting factor.
L.A.T.S.	Long-acting thyroid stimulator.
L.H.	Luteinising hormone.
L.H.R.F.	Luteinising-hormone releasing factor.
M.C.R.	Metabolic clearance-rate.
M.I.H.	Melanocyte-inhibiting factor.
mR.N.A.	Messenger R.N.A.
M.S.H.	Melanocyte-stimulating hormone.
N.A.D.P.	Nicotinamide adenine dinucleotide phosphate
P.B.I.	Protein-bound iodine.
P.I.F.	Prolactin-inhibiting factor.
R.F.	Releasing factor.
R.N.A.	Ribonucleic acid.
S.H.B.G.	Sex-hormone-binding globulin.
T3	Triiodothyronine.
T4	Thyroxine
T.B.G.	Thyroxine-binding globulin.
T.B.P.A.	Thyroxine-binding prealbumin.
Te B.G.	Testosterone-œstradiol binding globulin (also S.H.B.G.).
T.R.F.	*see* T.S.H.R.F.
T.S.H.	Thyroid-stimulating hormone.
T.S.H.R.F.	Thyroid-stimulating-hormone releasing factor.

Index

Figures in italics refer to illustrations.

Abortion, spontaneous, and
 human chorionic somato-
 mammotrophin, 26
Acromegaly, 21. 32, 38
 growth-hormone secretion in,
  34
 suppression tests for, 6
Addison's disease, 30
Adenosine monophosphate, cyclic,
 as second messenger, 3, *4*
 growth-hormone secretion and,
  30
 hormone action and, 2
Adenyl-cyclase system and
 hormone action, 2
Adrenal glands, 60–80
 disorders of, 73–80
 hyperplasia of, congenital, 79–80
 hypofunction of, stimulation
  tests for, 6
Adrenaline,
 action of, 3
 as insulin antagonist, 115
 growth-hormone secretion and,
  30
Adrenocorticotrophic hormone, 9
 action of, 2–3
 adrenal function and, 64–66,
  67
 assay of, 139
 control of, 10
 growth-hormone secretion and,
  30
 molecular weight, 17
 secretion of, by tumours, 7
 secretion-rate, 17
 structure of, 65, 66, *66*
Aldosterone,
 biosynthesis of, *61*

secretion of, control of, *68*,
 68–70
 secretion-rate, 71
Androgens,
 excess of, and hirsutism, 6
 growth-hormone secretion and,
  29
Angiotensin,
 assay, 139
 II, origin of, 1
 See also Renin-angiotensin
  system
Anorexia nervosa, 27
Antidiuretic hormone, 17, *18*,
 18–19
 action of, 3
 assay of, 139
 hypersecretion of, 19
 in diabetes insipidus, 19
 secretion of, by tumours, 7
Arginine-infusion test for growth
 hormone, 30–31
Arginine-vasopressin, *See* Antidiuretic hormone
Arginine-vasotocin, 18, *18*

Bioassay of hormones, 138
Breast development,
 human chorionic somato-
  mammotrophin and,
  26
 oxytocin and, 19

Calcitonin, 1, 7, 83, 98, 99–101,
 100, 102, 103, 104–105
Calcium homœostasis, 98–105
Carbohydrate metabolism and
 growth-hormone deficiency,
  22

Catecholamines and growth-
    hormone secretion, 30
Cell membrane and hormone
    action, 2
Central nervous system in anterior-
    pituitary control, 12–13
Cholecystokinin, 7
Clomiphene, 54, 56
Conn's syndrome, 77–79
    hypertension in, 6
    suppression tests for, 6
Contraception, hormonal, 56–58
Corpus luteum, 44, 45
    in pregnancy, 122, 124–126, *127*
Corticosteroid-binding globulin,
    71
Corticosteroids,
    as insulin antagonists, 115
    growth-hormone secretion and,
    30
Corticotrophin, *See*
    Adrenocorticotrophic
    hormone
Corticotrophin-releasing factor, 10,
    64–65
Cortisol, *See* Hydrocortisone
Cretinism, 95–96
Cushing's syndrome, 30, 72, 73–77
    suppression tests for, 6

Dehydroepiandrosterone, 7
    plasma-levels of, 71
Diabetes insipidus, 19
Diabetes mellitus, 117–120
    growth hormone and, 22
    in acromegaly, 115
    pregnancy and, 26
Dihydrotestosterone, 1, 7
Diiodotyrosine, 82, *82*, 85–86
Dwarfism, hypopituitary, 21, *34*,
    34–35

Environmental stimuli, responses
    to, 13
Exercise and growth hormone, 27

Fasting and growth-hormone
    secretion, 27

Feedback,
    negative, 5
    in pituitary control, 11–12, *12*
    positive, 6
Fertilisation, 44
Fetoplacental unit, functions of,
    129–132
Fetus, endocrine system of,
    132–133
First messenger, 3
Fluorimetric assay of hormones,
    140
Follicle-stimulating hormone, 9,
    49, *50*, *51*, 51–52
    carbohydrate content, 16
    measurement of, 46
    molecular weight, 17
    secretion-rate, 17
    spermatogenesis and, 42
Follicle-stimulating-hormone
    releasing factor, 10
Forebrain, neural connections of,
    with hypothalamus, 12–13

Gastrin, 1, 7
Gene transcription and hormone
    action, 4
Gigantism, 21, 37
Globus pallidus, neural
    connections of, with
    hypothalamus, 12–13
Glucagon, 7, 116
    action of, 3
    assay, 139
    secretion of, *111*
Glucocorticoid excess,
    hypothalamic lesion of, 6–7
Glucose,
    growth-hormone suppressibility
    and, 32
    homœostasis, 106–120
Glucose tolerance, 116–117
Goitre,
    endemic, 95–96
    toxic, 92–95
Gonadotrophins,
    assay, 139

control of, 10
gonad development and, 40
in infertility, 54–55
measurement of, 46
secretion of
  by tumours, 7
  effect of odour on, 13
Gonads,
  development of, 40
  functions of, 40–41
  hypofunction of, stimulation
    tests for, 6
Graves' disease, 92–95
Growth,
  disorders of, growth-hormone
    secretion in, 30
  regulation of, 21
  without growth hormone, 37–38
Growth hormone, 7, 9, 21–38
  actions of, 21–24
  assay of, 139
  bioassay of, 21, 22
  carbohydrate metabolism and,
    22
  control of, 10, 11
  deficiency of, isolated, 36
  diabetogenic action of, 22–23
  human,
    prolactin-like activity of, 23,
      25
    structure of, 24
  inactive, 36
  molecular weight of, 17
  pituitary content of, 24
  radioimmunoassay of, 26
  replacement therapy with, 5
  secretion of, 24–38, 28
    assessment of, 30–32
    by tumours, 7
    disorders of, 34–38
  secretion-rate, 17, 24
  species specificity of, 23–24
  storage of, 25
Growth-hormone releasing factor,
  10, 11, 25

Hirsutism and androgen excess, 6
Histamine, action of, 3

Homœostasis, 5
Hormones,
  action of, 2–4, 3, 4
  assay of, 137–147
  concentrations of, 1
  definition of, 1–2
  growth-hormone secretion and,
    29–30
  measurement of, 6, 8
  secretion-rates, 6
    determination of, 145–147
  specificity of, 2
Human chorionic gonadotrophin,
  128
Human chorionic
    somatomammotrophin, 26,
    129, 135
  abortion, spontaneous, and, 26
  in pituitary dwarfism, 35–36
  trophoblast function and, 26
Human growth hormone, See
    Growth hormone
Human placental lactogen, 7,
    25–26
  secretion of, by tumours, 7
  See also Human chorionic
    somatomammotrophin
Hydrocortisone,
  biosynthesis of, 61
  replacement therapy with, 5
  secretion-rate, 71
17-Hydroxycorticosteroids, assay
    of, 140
11-Hydroxylase deficiency, 79–80
17-Hydrooxylase deficiency, 80
21-Hydroxylase deficiency, 79
Hyperaldosteronism, 77–79
Hyperparathyroidism, 102–104
Hypertension in Conn's syndrome,
    6
Hyperthyroidism, 92–95
  growth-hormone secretion and,
    29
Hypoglycæmia, insulin-induced,
    26–27
  growth-hormone secretion and,
    30, 31, 32
Hypoparathyroidism, 103

Hypophysectomy, 21–22
Hypopituitarism, growth-hormone
    secretion in, *34*, 34–55
Hypothalamus,
    anterior-pituitary regulation
        and, 9–13, *12*, 14
    glucocorticoid excess and, 6–7
    hormones of, 7, 10–11
    in control of reproductive
        cycles, 14
    neural connections of, 12–13
    sexual differentiation of, 14
Hypothyroidism, 95–96

Implantation, 44–45
Imprinting, 13
Infertility, treatment of, 54–56
Inhibiting factors, 10
Insulin,
    action of, 3, 112–113
    assay, 139, 143
    biosynthesis, 108–109
    glucose homœostasis and,
        106–120
    secretion of, 109–112, *111*
    structure of, 107, *108*
Insulin antagonists, 114–115
Iodine metabolism, 84–85
Islets of Langerhans, 107, 116
Isotope derivative assay, 140

17-Ketosteroids,
    assay of, 140
    secretion-rates of, 71

Labour, oxytocin in, 19
Lactation, 26, 134–135
Leydig cells, 42, 43
Light and reproductive
    behaviour, 13
Limbic system, neural connections
    of, with hypothalamus,
    12–13
Lipotrophic hormone, 9
Long-acting thyroid stimulator,
    92–93

Lung tumours, hormone secretion
    by, 7
Luteinising hormone, 9, *49, 50,
    51*, 51–52
    action of, 3
    carbohydrate content of, 16
    measurement of, 46
    molecular weight of, 17
    secretion-rate, 17
Luteinising-hormone releasing
    factor, 10, 11
Lysine-vasopressin, 18, *18*

Malnutrition, growth-hormone
    levels in, 27
Mammary-gland development,
    human chorionic
        somatomammotrophin and,
        26
    oxytocin and, 19
Mass detection in steroid assay,
    140
Melanocyte-inibiting factor, 10
Melanocyte-stimulating hormone,
    3, 9
    inhibition of, by hypothalamus,
        9
Melatonin and effect of light on
    reproduction, 13
Menstrual cycle, 5, 14, 43–44, *47,
    47*–48, *49, 51*
Metabolism, hormone regulation
    of, 9
Milk-ejection reflex, 13, 19
Monoiodotyrosine, 82, *82*, 85–86
Mucoviscidosis, growth-hormone
    levels in, 27

Neural stimuli and growth-
    hormone secretion, 29
Neurohormones, hypothalamic,
    10
Neurophysin, 17

Odour and reproductive function,
    13
Œstradiol, 52

Œstrogens,
  growth-hormone secretion and,
    29
  in male, 42
Œstrus,
  control of, 14
  effect of odour on, 13
Ovary, 43–44
  effect of light on, 13
Ovulation, 44
  control of, 46–47
  effect of odour on, 13
  induction of, 54–56
Oxytocin, 17, *18*, 19
  assay of, 139

Pancreas and glucose
    homœostasis, 107
Parathormone,
  action of, 3
  calcium homœostasis and, 98,
    99, *100*, *102*, *103*
  secretion of, by tumours, 7
Parathyroid glands,
  calcium homœostasis and,
    98–104, *102*, *103*
  disorders of, 102–104
Parathyroid hormone, *See*
    Parathormone
Parturition, 134
Peptide hormones, concentrations
    of, 1
'Pergonal', 54
Pineal gland and effect of light on
    reproduction, 13
Pituitary gland, 9–19
  anterior,
    blood supply of, 9, 10
    cell types, 13–14
    central nervous system in
      control of, 12–13
    control of, 9–14, *10*
    growth regulation and, 21
    hormones of, 16–17
    secretory mechanism of, *15*
  hypofunction of, stimulation
      tests for, 6
  posterior, 17–19

Placenta,
  functions of, 130–132
  hormone secretion by, 122, *127*,
    128–129
Placental lactogen, *See* Human
    chorionic somatomammo-
    trophin
Porter-Silber reaction, 140
Pregnancy,
  effect of odour on, 13
  endocrine changes in, 122–135
Progestagens and hormone
    secretion, 29
Progesterone, 52
  in pregnancy, 125–128
  17α OH-Progesterone, *52*
Proinsulin, *108*
Prolactin, 9, 25, 135
  assay, 139
  inhibition of,
    by hypothalamus, 9
    by odour, 13
Prolactin-inhibiting factor, 10
Prostaglandins, 3
Protein-binding assay, 141–142
Pygmies, 36

Radioimmunoassay of hormones,
    143–145, *145*
Receptor sites, 2
Releasing factors, 10
Renin-angiotensin system, 1,
    69–70, *70*
Replacement therapy, 5
Reproduction, 40–58
  environmental stimuli and, 13
  hormone regulation of, 9
  light and, 13
  odour and, 13

Saturation analysis, 141–142
Second messenger, 3
Secretin, 1, 7
Serotonin, 3
Sertoli cells, 41, 42
Sex-hormone-binding globulin, 71
Sex hormones and growth-
    hormone secretion, 29

Sexual behaviour,
    environmental stimuli and, 13
    hormonal control of, 123–124
Spermatogensis, 41–42
Spermatozoa, development of, 41
Starvation and growth-hormone
    secretion, 27
Steroid hormones, *3*
    adrenal, 60–64, *61*
    action of, *3*
    assay of, 73
    biological effects of, 62–63
    biosynthesis of, 63–64
    metabolism of, 72
    regulation of, *66*
    secretion of, 61, 71–73
    disorders of, 73–80
    transport of, 71–73
    assay of, 140, *141*
    as third messenger, 3–4
    concentrations of, 1
    gonadal, action of, 1
    biosynthesis of, *41*
Stimulation tests for endocrine
    hypofunction, 6
Stress,
    growth-hormone secretion and,
    28
    neuroendocrine response to, 13
Suppression tests for endocrine
    hypersecretion, 6
'Synacthen', 66

Testis, 41–43
Testosterone, 42–43
    origin of, 1
Testosterone-œstradiol-binding
    globulin, 71
Tetraiodothyronine, *See*
    Thyroxine
Third messenger, 3–4
Thyroglobulin, 82, 84, 85, 86
Thyroid gland, 82–96, *87*
    C cells, 83
    disorders of, 92–96
    evolution of, 82, 83
    hypofunction of, tests for, 6

Thyroid hormones, concentrations
    of, 1
Thyroid-stimulating hormone, 9,
    84, 85, 86–89
    actions of, 3, 88–89
    assay of, 139
    control of, 10
    molecular weight, 17
    radioimmunoassay of, 89
    secretion-rate, 17
Thyroid-stimulating-hormone
    releasing factor, 10, 11,
    86–88
Thyrotoxicosis, 7, 92–95
    suppression tests for, 6
Thryotrophin, *See* Thyroid-
    stimulating hormone
Thyrotrophin-releasing factor,
    See Thyroid-stimulating-
    hormone releasing factor
Thyroxine, *82*
    action of, 3
    assay of, 90
    growth-hormone secretion and,
    25, 29
    iodine content of, 90
    metabolism of, 90–91
    replacement therapy with, 5
    synthesis, 85–86
Transcortin, *See* Corticosteroid-
    binding globulin
Triiodothyronine, *82*
    metabolism of, 90–91
    synthesis of, 85–86
Trophic hormones, 1, 5, 9
Tumours, hormone secretion by, 7

Ultimobranchial body, 83

Vasopressin, *See* Antidiuretic
    hormone
Vasotocin, 18
Vitamin D and calcium
    homœostasis, 98, 101–102,
    102, 103

Zimmerman reaction, 140